Bone Development and Disease in Infants

Bone Development and Disease in Infants

Editor

Vito Pavone

MDPI • Basel • Beijing • Wuhan • Barcelona • Belgrade • Manchester • Tokyo • Cluj • Tianjin

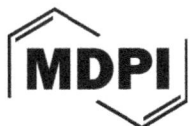

Editor
Vito Pavone
Department of General
Surgery and Medical Surgical
Specialties, University of
Catania, 95123 Catania, Italy
Policlinico Universitario
Catania
Catania
Italy

Editorial Office
MDPI
St. Alban-Anlage 66
4052 Basel, Switzerland

This is a reprint of articles from the Special Issue published online in the open access journal *Children* (ISSN 2227-9067) (available at: www.mdpi.com/journal/children/special_issues/Bone_Disease_Infants).

For citation purposes, cite each article independently as indicated on the article page online and as indicated below:

LastName, A.A.; LastName, B.B.; LastName, C.C. Article Title. *Journal Name* **Year**, *Volume Number*, Page Range.

ISBN 978-3-0365-4046-7 (Hbk)
ISBN 978-3-0365-4045-0 (PDF)

© 2022 by the authors. Articles in this book are Open Access and distributed under the Creative Commons Attribution (CC BY) license, which allows users to download, copy and build upon published articles, as long as the author and publisher are properly credited, which ensures maximum dissemination and a wider impact of our publications.

The book as a whole is distributed by MDPI under the terms and conditions of the Creative Commons license CC BY-NC-ND.

Contents

Preface to "Bone Development and Disease in Infants" vii

Vito Pavone
Bone Development and Disease in Infants
Reprinted from: *Children* 2022, 9, 519, doi:10.3390/children9040519 1

Daniela Dibello, Marcella Salvemini, Carlo Amati, Antonio Colella, Giusi Graziano and Giovanni Vicenti et al.
Trauma in Children during Lockdown for SARS-CoV-2 Pandemic. A Brief Report
Reprinted from: *Children* 2021, 8, 1131, doi:10.3390/children8121131 3

Lorenzo Moretti, Davide Bizzoca, Claudio Buono, Teresa Ladogana, Federica Albano and Biagio Moretti
Sports and Children with Hemophilia: Current Trends
Reprinted from: *Children* 2021, 8, 1064, doi:10.3390/children8111064 9

Vito Pavone, Andrea Vescio, Annalisa Culmone, Alessia Caldaci, Piermario La Rosa and Luciano Costarella et al.
Interobserver Reliability of Pirani and Dimeglio Scores in the Clinical Evaluation of Idiopathic Congenital Clubfoot
Reprinted from: *Children* 2021, 8, 618, doi:10.3390/children8080618 17

Carmine Zoccali, Silvia Careri, Dario Attala, Michela Florio, Giuseppe Maria Milano and Marco Giordano
A New Proximal Femur Reconstruction Technique after Bone Tumor Resection in a Very Small Patient: An Exemplificative Case
Reprinted from: *Children* 2021, 8, 442, doi:10.3390/children8060442 25

Vito Pavone, Andrea Vescio, Alessia Caldaci, Annalisa Culmone, Marco Sapienza and Mattia Rabito et al.
Sport Ability during Walking Age in Clubfoot-Affected Children after Ponseti Method: A Case-Series Study
Reprinted from: *Children* 2021, 8, 181, doi:10.3390/children8030181 33

Maurizio De Pellegrin, Chiara Maria Damia, Lorenzo Marcucci and Desiree Moharamzadeh
Double Diapering Ineffectiveness in Avoiding Adduction and Extension in Newborns Hips
Reprinted from: *Children* 2021, 8, 179, doi:10.3390/children8030179 41

Abel Emanuel Moca, Luminița Ligia Vaida, Rahela Tabita Moca, Anamaria Violeta Țuțuianu, Călin Florin Bochiș and Sergiu Alin Bochiș et al.
Chronological Age in Different Bone Development Stages: A Retrospective Comparative Study
Reprinted from: *Children* 2021, 8, 142, doi:10.3390/children8020142 49

Ho-Seok Oh, Myung-Jin Sung, Young-Min Lee, Sungmin Kim and Sung-Taek Jung
Does the Duration of Each Waldenström Stage Affect the Final Outcome of Legg–Calvé–Perthes Disease Onset before 6 Years of Age?
Reprinted from: *Children* 2021, 8, 118, doi:10.3390/children8020118 57

Vito Pavone, Claudia de Cristo, Andrea Vescio, Ludovico Lucenti, Marco Sapienza and Giuseppe Sessa et al.
Dynamic and Static Splinting for Treatment of Developmental Dysplasia of the Hip: A Systematic Review
Reprinted from: *Children* 2021, 8, 104, doi:10.3390/children8020104 63

Alexandru Herdea, Alexandru Ulici, Alexandra Toma, Bogdan Voicu and Adham Charkaoui
The Relationship between the Dominant Hand and the Occurrence of the Supracondylar Humerus Fracture in Pediatric Orthopedics
Reprinted from: *Children* **2021**, *8*, 51, doi:10.3390/children8010051 . . . . **75**

Andrea Vescio, Gianluca Testa, Annalisa Culmone, Marco Sapienza, Fabiana Valenti and Fabrizio Di Maria et al.
Treatment of Complex Regional Pain Syndrome in Children and Adolescents: A Structured Literature Scoping Review
Reprinted from: *Children* **2020**, *7*, 245, doi:10.3390/children7110245 . . . . **81**

Preface to "Bone Development and Disease in Infants"

Children's bone growth is continuous, and remodelling is always extensive. Growth proceeds from a vulnerable part of the bone, the growth plate. In remodelling, old bone tissue is gradually replaced by new tissue. Many bone disorders arise from the changes that occur in a growing child's musculoskeletal system, and these disorders can positively or negatively impact bone development. Other bone disorders may be inherited or occur in childhood for unknown reasons.

Bone disorders in children can result from factors that affect people of all ages, including injury, infection (osteomyelitis), cancer, and metabolic diseases. Causes of bone disorders can involve the gradual misalignment of bones and stress on growth plates during growth. Congenital deformities such as clubfoot or developmental dysplasia of the hip can lead to important alterations of bone development, causing severe dysfunction. Certain rare connective tissue disorders can also affect the bones, such as Marfan syndrome, osteogenesis imperfecta, and osteochondrodysplasias.

Many specialists are involved in the management of bone development disorders in children and adolescents, such as neurosurgeons, plastic surgeons, general surgeons, ORL surgeons, maxillofacial surgeons, orthopaedics, radiologists, and pediatric intensive care physicians.

The aim of this Special Issue is to present the latest research on the etiology, physiopathology, diagnosis and screening, management, and rehabilitation related to bone development and disease in infants, focusing on congenital, developmental, post-traumatic, and post-infective disorders.

Vito Pavone
Editor

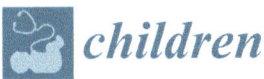

Editorial

Bone Development and Disease in Infants

Vito Pavone

Department of General Surgery and Medical Surgical Specialties, Section of Orthopaedics and Traumatology, A.O.U. Policlinico Rodolico—San Marco, University of Catania, 95123 Catania, Italy; vitopavone@hotmail.com

The aim of this Editorial is to introduce the content of the present Special Issue, entitled "Bone Development and Disease in Infants". Over the years, the orthopedic management of children affected by bone diseases has seen numerous changes, thanks to the continuous scientific confrontation and advances. It is therefore fundamental to keep on researching and exchanging ideas and results, aiming to give the best chances possible to our little patients. For this reason, this Special Issue represents a wonderful occasion since it provides a picture of today's knowledge and creates a collective discussion on the hot topics of pediatric orthopedics. From trauma to congenital and developmental disease, to the analysis of normal bone development, this Special Issue presents a selection of eleven outstanding articles, chosen carefully for our readers from numerous valid manuscripts. These articles are very interesting and constitute valid ground for everyone in the field.

The collection starts with the latest research works on a timeless topic: clubfoot. In the first communication, the analysis of the reliability of Pirani and Dimeglio scores in different medical figures (from residents to orthopedic surgeons) provides a picture of two solid evaluation methods that can be used widely by the medical community, especially for congenital talipes equinovarus [1]. Then, another selected manuscript regarding clubfoot analyzes sport ability during walking age following the Ponseti method: once again, it proves to be a valid therapeutic tool for these little patients [2].

Moving to another congenital orthopedic disease, developmental dysplasia of the hip, a group of colleagues underline the ineffectiveness of double diapering in its treatment [3]. In addition, it was decided to include a systematic review on this topic, in order to clarify DDH treatment options. This review analyzes dynamic and static splint differences, explaining the correct indication for the use of one or the other [4]. These first four articles question old standardized methods of diagnosis and treatment, confirming that the most used methods still represent the first choice.

In terms of more general topics, Moca et al. conducted an interesting retrospective comparative study on chronological age in different bone development stages by using lateral cephalometric radiographs and the cervical vertebral maturation method, adding useful information about bone growth and its stages [5]. Another classification was questioned in the article by Oh et al., where the duration of the Waldenström stage was used to evaluate early-onset Legg–Calvè–Perthes disease and its correlation with conservative treatment outcomes [6].

Moreover, two other reviews are included in this Special Issue. One is an analysis of sports and children with hemophilia that exhaustively assesses the actual trends in these patients' care and everyday life [7], and the other review investigates the literature concerning the treatment of complex regional pain syndrome in children and adolescents, offering tools on how to handle these cases [8].

Between the different articles, a case report was selected for this collection, which is always useful to readers who can find ideas and stimuli for their own difficult cases. Zoccali et al. display a case of a brilliant proximal femur reconstruction after bone tumor resection in an infant patient [9].

It was only right to present a piece on pediatric trauma: one article studied the correlation between the dominant hand and supracondylar humerus fracture, suggesting

Citation: Pavone, V. Bone Development and Disease in Infants. *Children* **2022**, *9*, 519. https://doi.org/10.3390/children9040519

Received: 22 December 2021
Accepted: 23 December 2021
Published: 6 April 2022

Publisher's Note: MDPI stays neutral with regard to jurisdictional claims in published maps and institutional affiliations.

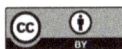

Copyright: © 2022 by the author. Licensee MDPI, Basel, Switzerland. This article is an open access article distributed under the terms and conditions of the Creative Commons Attribution (CC BY) license (https://creativecommons.org/licenses/by/4.0/).

that children probably tend to fall on their non-dominant hand to protect the dominant one [10].

The current pandemic could not go without discussion in this Special Issue, since our field has also been widely shaken by the ongoing SARS-CoV-2 pandemic that continues to affect our lives and those of our patients. Dibello et al. report differences in trauma in children during this unprecedented time, pointing out very interesting findings [11].

To conclude, I would like to thank the prestigious colleagues that helped me develop this Special Issue, analyzing a plethora of valid articles, and offering their best opinions. I hope this is going to be a pleasant read that can be helpful by adding useful information, widening readers' knowledge, and fueling the collective discussion on these selected topics.

Funding: This Editorial received no external funding.

Conflicts of Interest: The author declares no conflict of interest.

References

1. Pavone, V.; Vescio, A.; Culmone, A.; Caldaci, A.; Rosa, P.L.; Costarella, L.; Testa, G. Interobserver Reliability of Pirani and Dimeglio Scores in the Clinical Evaluation of Idiopathic Congenital Clubfoot. *Children* **2021**, *8*, 618. [CrossRef]
2. Pavone, V.; Vescio, A.; Caldaci, A.; Culmone, A.; Sapienza, M.; Rabito, M.; Canavese, F.; Testa, G. Sport Ability during Walking Age in Clubfoot-Affected Children after Ponseti Method: A Case-Series Study. *Children* **2021**, *8*, 181. [CrossRef] [PubMed]
3. De Pellegrin, M.; Damia, C.M.; Marcucci, L.; Moharamzadeh, D. Double Diapering Ineffectiveness in Avoiding Adduction and Extension in Newborns Hips. *Children* **2021**, *8*, 179. [CrossRef] [PubMed]
4. Pavone, V.; de Cristo, C.; Vescio, A.; Lucenti, L.; Sapienza, M.; Sessa, G.; Pavone, P.; Testa, G. Dynamic and Static Splinting for Treatment of Developmental Dysplasia of the Hip: A Systematic Review. *Children* **2021**, *8*, 104. [CrossRef] [PubMed]
5. Moca, A.E.; Vaida, L.L.; Moca, R.T.; Țuțuianu, A.V.; Bochiș, C.F.; Bochiș, S.A.; Iovanovici, D.C.; Negruțiu, B.M. Chronological Age in Different Bone Development Stages: A Retrospective Comparative Study. *Children* **2021**, *8*, 142. [CrossRef]
6. Oh, H.-S.; Sung, M.-J.; Lee, Y.-M.; Kim, S.; Jung, S.-T. Does the Duration of Each Waldenström Stage Affect the Final Outcome of Legg–Calvé–Perthes Disease Onset before 6 Years of Age? *Children* **2021**, *8*, 118. [CrossRef] [PubMed]
7. Moretti, L.; Bizzoca, D.; Buono, C.; Ladogana, T.; Albano, F.; Moretti, B. Sports and Children with Hemophilia: Current Trends. *Children* **2021**, *8*, 1064. [CrossRef] [PubMed]
8. Vescio, A.; Testa, G.; Culmone, A.; Sapienza, M.; Valenti, F.; Di Maria, F.; Pavone, V. Treatment of Complex Regional Pain Syndrome in Children and Adolescents: A Structured Literature Scoping Review. *Children* **2020**, *7*, 245. [CrossRef] [PubMed]
9. Zoccali, C.; Careri, S.; Attala, D.; Florio, M.; Milano, G.M.; Giordano, M. A New Proximal Femur Reconstruction Technique after Bone Tumor Resection in a Very Small Patient: An Exemplificative Case. *Children* **2021**, *8*, 442. [CrossRef] [PubMed]
10. Herdea, A.; Ulici, A.; Toma, A.; Voicu, B.; Charkaoui, A. The Relationship between the Dominant Hand and the Occurrence of the Supracondylar Humerus Fracture in Pediatric Orthopedics. *Children* **2021**, *8*, 51. [CrossRef] [PubMed]
11. Dibello, D.; Salvemini, M.; Amati, C.; Colella, A.; Graziano, G.; Vicenti, G.; Moretti, B.; Pederiva, F. Trauma in Children during Lockdown for SARS-CoV-2 Pandemic. A Brief Report. *Children* **2021**, *8*, 1131. [CrossRef]

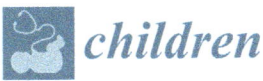

Brief Report

Trauma in Children during Lockdown for SARS-CoV-2 Pandemic. A Brief Report

Daniela Dibello [1,*], Marcella Salvemini [1], Carlo Amati [1], Antonio Colella [1], Giusi Graziano [2], Giovanni Vicenti [2], Biagio Moretti [2] and Federica Pederiva [3]

[1] Unit of Pediatric Orthopaedics and Traumatology Giovanni XXIII Children's Hospital, University of Bari, 70126 Bari, Italy; giannicaizzi@libero.it (M.S.); dr.carloamati@gmail.com (C.A.); colella31@gmail.com (A.C.)
[2] Orthopedic & Trauma Unit, Department of Basic Medical Sciences, Neuroscience and Sense Organs, School of Medicine, University of Bari Aldo Moro, 70124 Bari, Italy; giusi.graziano78@gmail.com (G.G.); dott.gvicenti@gmail.com (G.V.); biagio.moretti@uniba.it (B.M.)
[3] Pediatric Surgery Department, "Vittore Buzzi" Children's Hospital, 20154 Milano, Italy; federica.pederiva@asst-fbf-sacco.it
* Correspondence: daniela.dibello@policlinico.ba.it

Abstract: Purpose: The national lockdown established by the Italian government began on the 11th of March 2020 as a means to control the spread of SARS-CoV-2 infections. The purpose of this brief report is to evaluate the effect of the national lockdown on the occurrence and characteristics of trauma in children during lockdown. Methods: All children admitted to our paediatric orthopaedic unit with a diagnosis of fracture or trauma, including sprains and contusions, between 11 March 2020 and 11 April 2020, were retrospectively reviewed. Their demographic data, type of injury, anatomical location and need for hospitalisation were compared with the equivalent data of children admitted for trauma in the same period of 2018 and 2019. Results: Sixty-nine patients with trauma were admitted in 2020, with a significant decrease in comparison with 2019 ($n = 261$) and 2018 ($n = 289$) ($p < 0.01$). The patients were significantly younger, and the rate of fractures significantly increased in 2020 ($p < 0.01$). Conclusions: Home confinement decreased admissions to the emergency department for trauma by shutting down outdoor activities, schools and sports activities. However, the rate of fractures increased in comparison with minor trauma, involved younger children and had a worse prognosis.

Keywords: trauma; children; lockdown; pandemic; SARS-Co-V-2

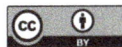

1. Introduction

The vast majority of paediatric injuries in emergency rooms are fractures, which are common during childhood [1,2] and are mostly caused by trauma while practising sports or playing [2]. Such injuries have a great impact on the child's and family's daily life and carry significant social and economic consequences, both in the short- and long term [1].

In an attempt to counteract the fast spread of the infection caused by SARS-CoV-2, the Italian government declared a national lockdown on the 9 March 2020 with consequent closure of schools, gymnasiums and all commercial and industrial activities, except for those deemed essential [3,4].

This is a brief report outlining the effects of the national lockdown on the occurrence and characteristics of trauma seen in children, comparing first aid access in our hospital from 11 March to 11 April in 2018, 2019 and 2020 (the hardest restriction period). Data in the same period for 2016 and 2017 were actually under investigation. Our main hypothesis was that the lockdown drastically reduced the total number of fractures in children and that only major traumas were brought to our attention at our second-level paediatric trauma centre.

2. Methods

After approval was received from the Institutional Research Committee, all children who came to our paediatric orthopaedic unit with a diagnosis of fracture or trauma, including sprains and contusions, between 11 March and 11 April 2020, were retrospectively reviewed. Demographic data, type of injury, anatomical location and the need for hospitalisation were recorded. Patients with polytrauma or with associated neurological impairment were excluded. Children admitted for fracture or trauma in the same interval of time in 2018 and 2019 were used as controls. The diagnosis was confirmed in all cases by physical examination and plain radiograph, without the need to perform a CT scan or MRI. The results were expressed as percentages or as means ± SD, and both groups were compared by nonparametric Mann–Whitney, chi-squared or Fisher tests, as appropriate, with a threshold of significance at $p < 0.05$. The analyses were performed using R software (version 3.5.2).

3. Results

Sixty-nine children (30 female and 39 male) presented during the study period in 2020 with a trauma involving the upper limb in 68%(n = 47), the lower limb in 28% (n = 19) and the spine in 4% (n = 3) of the cases. In the correspondent period in 2019, 260 children (100 female and 160 male) were treated for trauma of the upper limb in 55% (n = 143) of the cases, the lower limb in 36% (n = 94) and the spine in 9% (n = 23). In 2018, 289 children (112 female and 177 male) were treated for trauma of the upper limb in 57% (n = 165) of the cases, the lower limb in 35% (n = 101) and the spine in 8% (n = 23). The mean age of the patients treated in the emergency department in 2020 (6.83 ± 4.06) was significantly lower when compared with 2019 (10.84 ± 4.23) and 2018 (9.95 ± 4.42; $p < 0.001$). In all cases, the number of patients admitted to our emergency room in 2020 was significantly lower than in 2019 and 2018 ($p < 0.001$).

In 2020, the number of fractures (29) was significantly higher in percentage in comparison with 2019 (67) and 2018 (68) when contusions and sprains were the most common lesions ($p < 0.01$) (Figure 1). On the other hand, although the need to admit the patient to the ward was similar across all years, the prognosis (as estimated by the orthopaedic surgeon who treated the patient in the emergency room) for the trauma was significantly worse in 2020 ($p < 0.05$) (Figure 2). While pain or functional diseases not related to trauma decreased in our paediatric orthopaedic unit, major trauma with complicated wounds, tendon involvement and other injuries that required a multidisciplinary evaluation increased ("other" in Figure 1). Nevertheless, the total number of trauma and injuries in 2020 decreased compared to 2019 and 2018.

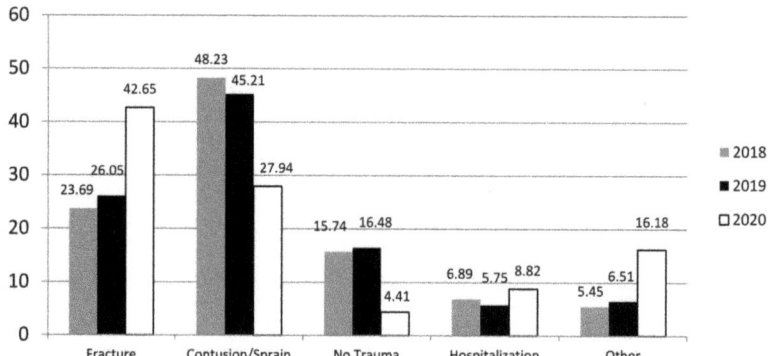

Figure 1. Comparison between 2018, 2019 and 2020 in terms of type of injury and need for hospitalization (in percentages).

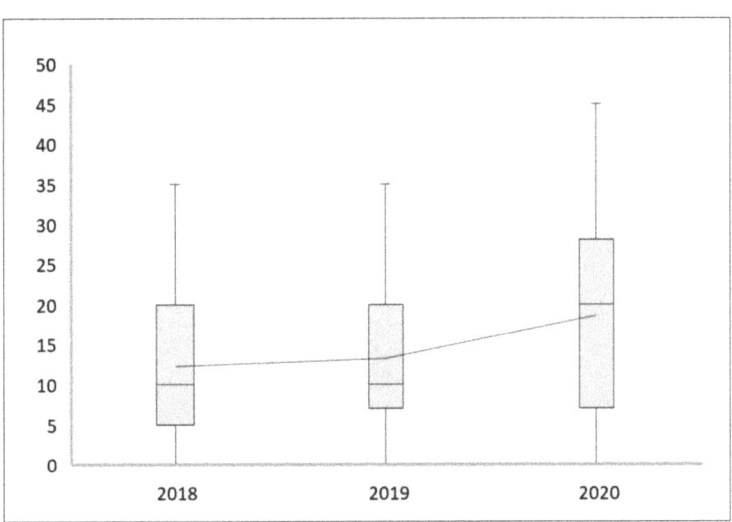

Figure 2. Comparison between 2018, 2019 and 2020 in terms of prognosis of the trauma.

In 2020, the trauma occurred mostly at home (83.6% n = 58) and sport-related injuries were significantly lower (16.4% n = 11) in comparison with 2019 (28.7% n = 75) and 2018 (29.8% n = 87). In 2019 and 2018, the trauma more frequently happened away from home and was not sport-related (42.7% n = 111 and 42.9% n = 124, respectively) but due to play-related activities. Of the remaining cases for 2019 and 2018, half occurred at home (28.7% n = 75 and 29.7% n = 86, respectively) and the other half (28.6% n = 74 and 27.3% n = 79, respectively) were sport-related (Figure 3). However, no significant differences were found when comparing 2018 and 2019 in terms of the type of injury, prognosis and location of the trauma.

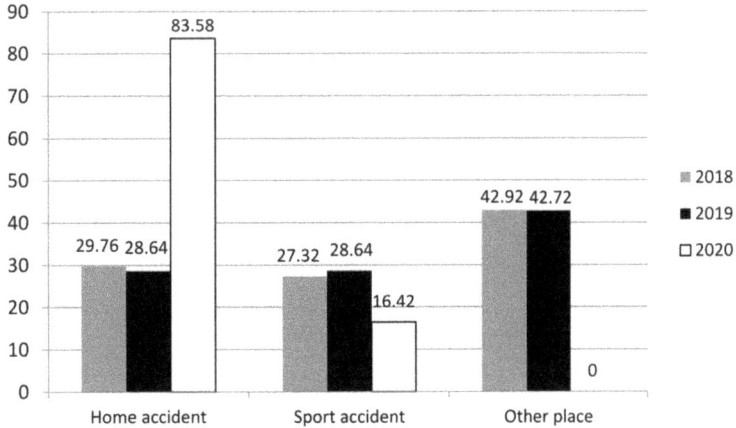

Figure 3. Comparison between 2018, 2019 and 2020 in terms of place in which trauma occurred (in percentages).

4. Discussion

Twelve percent of the admissions per year to the paediatric emergency department are due to musculoskeletal injuries [2,5]. The vast majority of these injuries are skeletal fractures, which cause significant morbidity to children and are an expensive public health issue. The overall rate of fractures is increasing despite the implementation of guidelines to prevent injuries and the campaign to raise parents' awareness of the subject [2,6,7].

The Italian national lockdown from the 11 March 2020 meant children spent most of their time indoors and were not allowed to practice outdoor sports or activities. The first outcome of the stay-at-home order was a significant decrease in admissions (76% less in comparison with 2019, and 77% in comparison with 2018) to the emergency department for trauma. Moreover, trauma usually happening at school or practising sports almost disappeared during the lockdown. Most of the trauma in 2020 occurred at home, while in 2019 and 2018, they mostly happened outdoor while playing. This result highlights how significantly sports and play impact the incidence of fractures in children.

The patients treated in 2020 were significantly younger than the ones seen in 2019 and 2018. One explanation is that the lockdown eliminated all the trauma occurring during school time or related to sports. During this time, older children, now staying at home, spent more time playing videogames, watching TV or following lessons online, whereas preschool-aged children did not change their activities at home, such as running or jumping up and down from couches and beds. This could explain why the percentage of the age of trauma is inversed in 2020 in comparison to 2019 and 2018.

The rate of fractures increased in percentage in 2020 and the prognosis using days of hospitalisation worsened. This data could be explained by the fact that parents preferred to treat minor traumas at home without visiting a hospital for diagnosis and treatment. The distribution of the site of fractures was not modified by the lockdown, and upper limb fractures continued to be the most usual ones at both endpoints. Forearm fractures are the most common ones in children, accounting for 40–50% of all fractures during childhood [1,8–10]. The distal third of the forearm, including the radius and/or ulna, is involved in 75% of the cases [11,12] because of the increased body mass during their growth and development together with decreased bone mineral content [5,6,9,11].

Our results were consistent with the finding of other groups [13–22], although only a few of them analysed a paediatric population. Our study, in fact, demonstrates how a lockdown could differently affect children according to the age group.

These data lead to several considerations: as previously said, during the lockdown, a lot of minor traumas were likely treated at home without reaching a hospital or calling for medical care. In this scenario, a hypothesis is that many children were treated with only analgesics and rest at home. In the future, to limit the access to a second-level trauma care hub, children with minor trauma (e.g., the frequent torus fractures of the distal radius) could be treated in a first-level emergency spot where alternatives to a plaster cast treatment could be used (especially if an orthopaedic specialist is not available). In this way, we are conducting a study about the efficacy of treating children with torus distal radius fractures with an easy-to-use 3D-printed splint in place of the classic plaster cast usually moulded by an orthopaedic specialist and a dedicated nurse. Results collected to date showed faster treatment in the emergency room, improved childhood activities during recovery and high satisfaction for parents and children without any complication or delay in the healing process as seen for splints in previous studies [23,24]. As we can easily expect new epidemic waves in the near future, changing medical care modalities for minor trauma in children (at the moment, the least vaccinated population) could improve our attempts to limit the spread of the virus.

Another consideration that could be extrapolated from these data is related to our experience in orthopaedic fast-tracking: in our hospital, in fact, after the nursing triage in the emergency room, children with uncomplicated monosegmental trauma are sent directly to our unit. Next, an orthopaedic surgeon evaluates the case, visits the child, requires radiographs and eventually CT scans and then decides for immobilisation or hospitalisation. In the first case, the patient is discharged directly home. This consolidated pathway, already described in the literature [25], demonstrates a shorter stay in the hospital, virtually no waiting time in an emergency room (where otherwise healthy children could be exposed to those with fevers, coughs or colds) and higher satisfaction for parents and children. In these months of worldwide strategies for containment efficiency and spread control for the COVID-19 pandemic, in our opinion, every attempt to reduce the risk of contagion should be pursued.

Notably, these considerations have limitations. First, we do not have data about a delay in treatment of fractures that do not reach a hospital soon after the trauma accident, and we did not collect data from other hospitals in our region that usually treat children from 12 to 18 years old, probably losing much of the data about fractures and treatments in this age range. We also did not consider weather patterns (March and April are usually lower-fracture-rate months compared to July or August), nor did we collect data about rainfalls and sunny days in 2018, 2019 and 2020. Lastly, we only considered rates of accidental trauma, which did not include any form of abuse, during the lockdown period.

5. Conclusions

In conclusion, home confinement decreased admissions to the emergency department for trauma by shutting down outdoor activities, schools and sports activities. The volume of paediatric patients seen for trauma during the lockdown decreased by about 75% from two years prior. Moreover, the patients who were seen during the lockdown were significantly younger children, probably because only children with major trauma were brought to the hospital by their parents to avoid exposure to the virus, whereas children with contusions and sprains were treated conservatively at home. This study finally demonstrates how a lockdown could differently affect children according to the age group.

Author Contributions: Study conception and design: D.D., F.P.; Data acquisition: M.S., A.C., C.A.; Analysis and data interpretation: M.S., A.C., C.A., G.G.; Drafting of the manuscript: D.D., F.P., C.A.; Critical revision: F.P., G.V., B.M. All authors have read and agreed to the published version of the manuscript.

Funding: This research received no external funding.

Institutional Review Board Statement: All procedures performed in studies involving human participants were in accordance with the ethical standards of the institutional and/or national research committee and with the 1964 Helsinki declaration and its later amendments or comparable ethical standards.

Informed Consent Statement: Informed consent was obtained from all individual participants included in the study.

Conflicts of Interest: The authors declare no conflict of interest.

References

1. Mamoowala, N.; Johnson, N.A.; Dias, J.J. Trends in paediatric distal radius fractures: An eight-year review from a large UK trauma unit. *Ann. R. Coll. Surg. Engl.* **2019**, *101*, 297–303. [CrossRef] [PubMed]
2. Segal, D.; Slevin, O.; Aliev, E.; Borisov, O.; Khateeb, B.; Faour, A.; Palmanovich, E.; Brin, Y.S.; Weigl, D. Trends in the seasonal variation of paediatric fractures. *J. Child. Orthop.* **2018**, *12*, 614–621. [CrossRef] [PubMed]
3. World Health Organization: Rolling Update on Coronavirus Disease (COVID 19). 2020. Available online: https://www.who.int/emergencies/diseass/novel-coronavirus2019/events-as-they-happen (accessed on 18 May 2021).
4. Prime Minister's Decree of 11 March 2020 "Iorestoacasa/Istayathome" (20A01558) (GU n.62 del 9-3-2020). Available online: https://www.gazzettaufficiale.it/gazzetta/serie_generale/caricaDettaglio?dataPubblicazioneGazzetta=2020-03-09&numeroGazzetta=62 (accessed on 18 May 2021).
5. Chamberlain, J.M.; Patel, K.M.; Pollack, M.M.; Brayer, A.; Macias, C.G.; Okada, P.; Schunk, J. Recalibration of the pediatric risk of admission score using a multi-institutional sample. *Ann. Emerg. Med.* **2004**, *43*, 461. [CrossRef]
6. Khosla, S.; Melton, L.J.; Dekutoski, M.B.; Achenbach, S.J.; Oberg, A.L.; Riggs, B.L. Incidence of childhood distal forearm fractures over 30 years: A population-based study. *JAMA* **2003**, *290*, 1479. [CrossRef]
7. Jones, I.E.; Williams, S.M.; Dow, N.; Goulding, A. How many children remain fracture-free during growth? A longitudinal study of children and adolescents participating in the Dunedin Multidisciplinary Health and Development Study. *Osteoporos. Int.* **2002**, *13*, 990. [CrossRef] [PubMed]
8. Price, C.T.; Flynn, J.M. Management of fractures. In *Lovell and Winter's Pediatric Orthopaedics*, 6th ed.; Morrissey, R.T., Weinstein, S.L., Eds.; Lippincott: Philadelphia, PA, USA, 2006; p. 1463.
9. Rodríguez-Merchán, E.C. Pediatric fractures of the forearm. *Clin. Orthop. Relat. Res.* **2005**, *432*, 65–72. [CrossRef]

10. Jones, I.E.; Cannan, R.; Goulding, A. Distal forearm fractures in New Zealand children: Annual rates in a geographically defined area. *N. Zeal. Med. J.* **2000**, *113*, 443.
11. Pizzutillo, P.D. Pediatric orthopaedics. In *Essentials of Musculoskeletal Care*, 3rd ed.; Griffin, Y.L., Ed.; American Academy of Orthopaedic Surgeons: Rosemont, IL, USA, 2005; p. 863.
12. Abraham, A.; Handoll, H.H.; Khan, T. Interventions for treating wrist fractures in children. *Cochrane Database Syst. Rev.* **2008**, *12*, CD004576.
13. Testa, G.; Sapienza, M.; Rabuazzo, F.; Culmone, A.; Valenti, F.; Vescio, A.; Pavone, V. Comparative study between admission, orthopaedic surgery, and economic trends during Covid-19 and non-Covid-19 pandemic in an Italian tertiary hospital: A retrospective review. *J. Orthop. Surg. Res.* **2021**, *16*, 1–11. [CrossRef] [PubMed]
14. Christey, G.; Amey, J.; Campbell, A.; Smith, A. Variation in volumes and characteristics of trauma patients admitted to a level one trauma centre during national level 4 lockdown for COVID-19 in New Zeland. *N. Zeal. Med. J.* **2020**, *133*, 81–88.
15. Hernigou, J.; Morel, X.; Callewier, A.; Bath, O.; Hernigou, P. Staying home during "Covid-19" decreased fractures, but trauma did not quarantine in one hundred and twelve adults and twenty eight children and the "tsunami of recommendations" could not lockdown twelve elective operations. *Int. Orthop.* **2020**, *44*, 1473–1480. [CrossRef]
16. Clementsen, S.; Randsborg, P.H. School related fractures. *Tidsskr. Nor. Laegeforen* **2014**, *134*, 521–524. [CrossRef] [PubMed]
17. Del Papa, J.; Vittorini, P.; D'Aloisio, F.; Muselli, M.; Giuliani, A.R.; Mascitelli, A.; Fabiani, L. Retrospective Analysis of Injuries and Hospitalizations of Pazients Followig the 2009 Earthquake of L'Aquila City. *Int. J. Environ. Res. Public Health* **2019**, *16*, 1675. [CrossRef] [PubMed]
18. Nabian, M.H.; Vosoughi, F.; Najafi, F.; Khabiri, S.S.; Nafisi, M.; Veisi, J.; Rastgou, V.; Ghamari, S.; Aakhashi, A.; Bahrami, N.; et al. Epidemiological pattern of pediatric trauma in COVID-19 outbreak: Data from a tertiary trauma center in Iran. *Injury* **2020**, *51*, 2811–2815. [CrossRef] [PubMed]
19. Bram, J.T.; Johnson, M.A.; Magee, L.C.; Mehta, N.N.; Fazal, F.Z.; Baldwin, K.D.; Riley, J.; Shah, A.S. Where have all the fractures gone? The epidemiology of pediatric fractures during the COVID-19 Pandemic. *J. Pediatr. Orthop.* **2020**, *40*, 373–379. [CrossRef] [PubMed]
20. Dolci, A.; Marongiu, G.; Leinardi, L.; Lombardo, M.; Dessì, G.; Capone, A. The epidemiology of fractures and muskulo-skeletal traumas during COVID-19 lockdown: A detailed survey of 17.591 patients in a wide Italian metropolitan area. *Geriatr. Orthop. Surg. Rehabil.* **2020**, *11*, 2151459320972673. [CrossRef] [PubMed]
21. Rajput, K.; Sud, A.; Rees, M.; Rutka, O. Epidemiology of trauma presentations to a major trauma centre in the North West of England during the COVID-19 level 4 lockdown. *Eur. J. Trauma Emerg. Surg.* **2021**, *47*, 631–636. [CrossRef]
22. Chiba, H.; Lewis, M.; Benjamin, E.R.; Jakob, D.A.; Liasidis, P.; Wong, M.D.; Navarrete, S.; Carreon, R.; Demetriades, D. "Safer at home": The effect of the COVID-19 lockdown on epidemiology, resource utilization, and outcomes at a large urban trauma center. *J. Trauma Acute Care Surg.* **2021**, *90*, 708. [CrossRef] [PubMed]
23. Neal, E. Comparison of splinting and casting in the management of torus fracture. *Emerg. Nurse* **2014**, *21*, 22–26. [CrossRef] [PubMed]
24. Williams, B.A.; Alvarado, C.A.; Montoya-Williams, D.C.; Matthias, R.C.; Blakemore, L.C. Buckling down on torus fractures: Has evolving evidence affected practice? *J. Child. Orthop.* **2018**, *12*, 123–128. [CrossRef] [PubMed]
25. Manno, E.; Pesce, M.; Stralla, U.; Festa, F.; Geninatti, S.; Balzarro, M.F.; Di Leo, D.; Gelain, B. Specialized fast track: A sustainable model to improve emergency department patient flow. *J. Hosp. Adm.* **2015**, *4*, 40. [CrossRef]

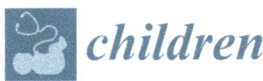

Review

Sports and Children with Hemophilia: Current Trends

Lorenzo Moretti [1], Davide Bizzoca [2,*], Claudio Buono [1], Teresa Ladogana [1], Federica Albano [1] and Biagio Moretti [1]

1. Orthopaedics Unit, Department of Basic Medical Science, Neuroscience and Sensory Organs, School of Medicine, University of Bari "Aldo Moro", AOU Consorziale Policlinico, 70124 Bari, Italy; lorenzo.moretti@libero.it (L.M.); claudio.buono@uniba.it (C.B.); teresa.ladogana@uniba.it (T.L.); federica.albano@uniba.it (F.A.); biagio.moretti@uniba.it (B.M.)
2. PhD Course in Public Health, Clinical Medicine and Oncology, University of Bari "Aldo Moro", Piazza Giulio Cesare 11, 70124 Bari, Italy
* Correspondence: da.bizzoca@gmail.com or davide.bizzoca@uniba.it

Abstract: Hemophilia is a sex-linked recessive disorder characterized by a lack of blood factors necessary for clotting. This review aims to investigate the benefits of sports activities in children with hemophilia in terms of both physical and psychological wellness. Sports activity is necessary for children with hemophilia to preserve joints' range of motion, reduce joint bleeding, improve muscle mass and strength, enhance proprioception and prevent secondary chronic diseases. In the past, high-impact sports were usually forbidden in children with hemophilia because of their high bleeding risk. Recent studies, however, have shown that prophylaxis therapy can allow a hemophilic child to take part in vigorous activities or high-impact sports. The benefits of sports activity in children with hemophilia are expressed by a better muscular trophism and an improved bone mineral density. Moreover, physical activity has a positive impact on children's psychosocial well-being. Due to prophylaxis therapy, the quality of life of children with hemophilia is similar to their peers, and this has allowed an improvement in sports participation, including team sports.

Keywords: hemophilia; children; sport; prophylaxis; high-impact sports; physical activity; psychological wellness

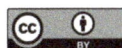

1. Introduction

Hemophilia is a sex-linked recessive disorder characterized by a lack of blood factors necessary for clotting [1].

This disease mainly occurs in males and the deficit may be in factor VIII (hemophilia type A or classic type) or factor IX (type B) [2]. Patients with severe plasma protein deficit can have recurrent muscular and especially joint bleeding episodes, which may lead to musculoskeletal pain and physical and functional ability reduction, thus finally compromising their quality of life [3].

Consequently, it is reported that hemophilic children tend to be more sedentary compared with non-hemophilic peers because of the difficulties they may experience during physical activity [4].

This review aims to investigate the benefits of sports activities in children with hemophilia in terms of both physical and psychological wellness.

2. Materials and Methods

The first step consisted of a scoping literature search performed by three reviewers, CB, TL and FA, supervised by DB, using the PubMed database to select an initial pool of potentially relevant papers, originally designed to investigate the feasibility of physical activity in children with hemophilia.

The search strategy included the following terms: ((hemophilia [MeSH Terms] OR "hemophilic patient" [All Fields]) OR (hemophilic child [MeSH Terms] OR "children with hemophilia" [All Fields])) AND ("sport" [MeSH Terms] OR (sport [All Fields]) OR "physical activity").

The second step consisted of revising the literature review to identify papers dealing with physical activity in children with hemophilia.

Inclusion criteria were: human studies in which the authors considered the role of sports activity in children affected by hemophilia; English language; studies about children with hemophilia.

A total of 42 articles [1,3–43] were finally included in the present review.

3. Hemophilia and Sports Participation

Sports activity is necessary for children with hemophilia to preserve joints' range of motion, reduce joint bleeding, improve muscle mass and strength, enhance proprioception and prevent secondary chronic diseases (i.e., cardiovascular disease, diabetes, cancer) [44]. To prevent joint and muscle bleeding, parents put their children with hemophilia through various exercise programs [5]. Muscle atrophy, instability and restriction of motion are the first visible signs of sedentarism [6], whereas early subclinical symptoms such as tender ligaments are found even in clinically healthy young people [1]. This leads to a lack of physical activity and exercise that results in a poor physical condition with diminished muscle strength, aerobic/anaerobic power, proprioception and flexibility [7]. Furthermore, sports activity can improve bone mineral density, which is lower in children with hemophilia than in healthy peers [8]. In the past, because of bleeding risk, sports activity was discouraged in children with chronic disease [9]. However, nowadays, due to new improvements in medical treatment, the participation of children with hemophilia in sport has improved [44].

However, even if an increase in participation in sports has been observed in children with hemophilia, aerobic activity is less practiced. This phenomenon may be explained considering that children with chronic diseases (such as cystic fibrosis or hemophilia) might have a decline in pulmonary function, which finally leads to less exercise tolerance [10]. Sports and exercise help to develop fundamental abilities, such as coordination, strength, endurance and flexibility. The muscle-to-fat ratio is improved, and, in the long term, joints are protected and bleeding episodes avoided [11].

Prophylaxis is effective to maintain a minimum level of clotting factor activity and to permit regular sports participation in children with hemophilia [12]. However, prophylaxis alone is insufficient to protect from bleeding and joint damage [13]. In fact, in children with hemophilia, it is important to maintain weight within a healthy range to prevent an overload of the joints, especially the knees and ankle [14]. Furthermore, sports exercise increases factor VIII levels and could modify coagulation parameters in mild/moderate hemophilia [15]. It is therefore reported that an increased plasmatic lactate concentration, secondary to anaerobic exercises, for instance, may affect FVIII clearance, thus improving the patient's coagulation [1].

In the past, high-impact sports were usually prohibited in children with hemophilia due to the high risk of bleeding injuries [16]. In the 1970s, it was a common practice to discourage any type of sports because of the risk of bleeding episodes, but today, the participation in sports activities by hemophilic patients has improved, and physical activity is considered healthy for this type of patient [17] even if high-impact sports are still not recommended. Nowadays, on the other hand, different guidelines are available to regulate hemophilic patients' sports participation; hemophilia type and severity play a key role in the correct sports activity choice [18,19]. According to some hemophilia centers, the choice of activities should reflect individual basis such as: preference/interest, ability, physical condition and resources [7]. Participation in non-contact sports (swimming, running and walking) should always be promoted, but high-impact sports (rugby, boxing, football and basketball) or sports such as motocross (endowed with a higher injury risk) are often discouraged even on good prophylactic therapy [7,11].

In the United States, the National Hemophilia Foundation (NHF) proposes the stratification of activities into safe, safe-to-moderate, moderate, moderate-to-dangerous and dangerous risk groups. The safe through moderate categories can be routinely recommended with the proper preparation [20]. Another stratification in high-impact and low-impact sport was proposed by Ross and Goldenberg in 2009: high-impact sports include soccer, basketball, baseball, bowling, gymnastics, field hockey, running, skiing, snowboarding, soccer, softball, tennis and track and field, while low-impact activities include weight training, cycling, Frisbee, golf, swimming and walking/hiking [21].

However, is it right to forbid children with hemophilia to participate in high-impact sports even if they are on prophylactic treatment?

According to some authors, prophylactic therapy can allow a hemophilic child to engage in vigorous activities or high-impact sports [44]. An article by Ross et al. [21] showed that children with hemophilia on prophylaxis could participate without any increased risk of joint bleedings.

The American Academy of Pediatrics (AAP) Committee on Sports Medicine and Fitness has divided childhood activities according to risks and formulated guidelines for sports participation [22]. The AAP has recommended that children should engage in trampoline activities only in professionally supervised settings due to the high risk of fractures, hospitalization and risk of bruises and other injuries [23]. For the same reason, no children should participate in boxing because this activity encourages injuries especially to the head and neck [24]. Additionally, the dangers of concussion related to US football and soccer have recently received attention, with recommendations for carefully monitoring children after an event [25]. Nonetheless, the AAP recommends participation in sports activities for children with bleeding disorders [21].

In 2017, the National Hemophilia Foundation (NHF) proposed some guidelines for athletic participation by patients with a bleeding disorder [20]. Therefore, a minimum of 60 min of exercise per day, with appropriate supervision, is recommended for children after receiving prophylaxis.

4. Treatment of Sports Injuries in Children with Hemophilia

Significant bleeding episodes in hemophilic patients are typically treated with the administration of missing clotting factors (factor VIII or IX), whereas they could be managed by bypassing agents or antifibrinolytic medication [1]. Missing factors should be administrated to permit regular sports activities in children with hemophilia with a severe deficiency (when the factors activity is lower than 10–20%) [27]. The high adherence in young children is related to the benefits of sports activity also without parents' supervision [26,45–49]. Non-adherence to prophylaxis could be responsible for an increase in joint bleeding, reduced quality of life and absence from school. Children should receive regular infusions to reduce the risk of bleeding to preserve joint wellness [28]. An alternative treatment, in the case of minor bleeding episodes, is the use of desmopressin (intravenously or intranasally) [1]. A study published in 1980 showed that desmopressin also increases factor VII plasma concentrations through the release of VWF (Von Willebrand Factor) [29]. The main complication after treatment with clotting factor concentrates is the development of inhibiting antibodies directed against some parts of factor VIII/IX, and these are the cause of a reduction in its coagulant activity [30]. Usually, inhibitors are produced in children within the first 50 days of treatment and they are the cause of an increase in the risk of bleeding episodes [31]. In the past, the usage of plasma, containing clotting factors, from unscreened donors made the transmission of blood viruses easier (HBV, HCV and HIV). Nowadays, donors are tested before blood donation [1].

5. Bleeding Prevention in Hemophilic Children

In children with lower (5% or less) factor levels, a higher bleeding risk has been observed during sports activity. It is reported that an increase of 1% in the factor level with treatment before sport correlates with a decreased bleeding risk by 2% [32,38–43].

Assessments of joint and muscle function before sport selection in children with hemophilia are required [33]. In addition, they require a complete evaluation, which should include: an analysis of balance and coordination, aerobic capacity and body fat content [23]. Although the risk of injury cannot be eliminated, protective measures can be taken to reduce the risk of injury: the use of helmets, facemasks, shin guards, kneepads, wrist and forearm guards according to the type of sports activity [34]. The risk of serious bleeding and the number of hemorrhages can be radically decreased with the use of prophylaxis with factor VIII and IX concentrates [21].

A higher factor level at the time of injury is a predictive factor of bleeding events. These observations offer the opportunity to minimize bleeding risks during participation in sports [35,50–53]. A way to reduce the risk of bleeding is to divide the dose of the prophylactic factor by the number of days per week and concerning sports participation [23]. In such a way, the factor level at the time of collision may be increased, reducing the risk of bleeding episodes [12,25,54–56].

Newer longer-acting clotting factors may improve the maintenance of a factor level enough to prevent bleeding. In addition, strengthening and warming up before sports participation may reduce the rate of sports injuries. The risk of participation in collision sports is only moderately increased in hemophilic boys in prophylactic therapy, so the risk of sports injuries in hemophilia becomes similar to that of their healthy peers [36,37].

6. Psychosocial Well-Being and Sports Activity

The positive impact of sports activity on psychosocial well-being is well known, and some studies have recently investigated the relationship between physical activity and the psychosocial dimension in hemophilic patients.

Von Macksen et al. [57], in a multicenter, cross-sectional study, have recently described the impact of sport on health-related quality of life (HRQoL), physical performance and clinical outcomes in adult patients affected by hemophilia. The authors recruited fifty hemophilic patients with mild ($n = 12$), moderate ($n = 10$) or severe ($n = 28$) hemophilia A (70%) or B (30%). Among the recruited patients, 36% of participants reported not participating in any sport, mainly because of their physical condition, whereas the remaining 64% of participants reported undertaking sporting activity, including high-impact sports. The authors showed that patients participating in more sport reported significantly better HRQoL than those participating in less sport ($p < 0.005$).

Similar findings were reported by Sondermann et al. [47] in hemophilic children. These authors showed that the increase in physical activity did not correlate with an increase in bleeding events in the recruited children. Moreover, a positive impact on the children's quality of life and participation in social/school activities was observed.

7. Conclusions

The benefits of sports activity in children with hemophilia are expressed by a better muscular trophism and an improved bone mineral density. Moreover, physical activity has a positive impact on children's psychosocial well-being.

Due to prophylaxis therapy, the quality of life of children with hemophilia is similar to their peers and this has allowed an improvement in sports participation, including team sports. While in the past, due to the high risk of injuries, participation especially in team sports had been discouraged, nowadays sports activity has been promoted to achieve better physical and social wellness.

Author Contributions: Conceptualization, L.M., D.B. and B.M.; validation, L.M., D.B. and B.M.; data curation, C.B., T.L. and F.A.; writing—original draft preparation, C.B., T.L. and F.A.; writing—review and editing, D.B.; visualization, L.M.; supervision, D.B.; project administration, B.M.; funding acquisition, B.M. All authors have read and agreed to the published version of the manuscript.

Funding: This research was supported by the University of Bari "Aldo Moro".

Institutional Review Board Statement: Not applicable.

Informed Consent Statement: Not applicable.

Data Availability Statement: Not applicable.

Conflicts of Interest: The authors declare no conflict of interest.

References

1. Fijnvandraat, K.; Cnossen, M.H.; Leebeek, F.W.G.; Peters, M. Diagnosis and management of haemophilia. *BMJ* **2012**, *344*, e2707. [CrossRef]
2. Knobe, K.; Berntorp, E. Haemophilia and Joint Disease: Pathophysiology, Evaluation, and Management. *J. Comorbidity* **2011**, *1*, 51–59. [CrossRef]
3. Azab, A.R.; Elnaggar, R.K.; Diab, R.H.; Moawd, S.A. Therapeutic value of kinesio taping in reducing lower back pain and improving back muscle endurance in adolescents with hemophilia. *J. Musculoskelet. Neuronal Interact.* **2020**, *20*, 256–264.
4. Takken, T.; Stephens, S.; Balemans, A.; Tremblay, M.S.; Esliger, D.; Schneiderman, J.; Biggar, D.; Longmuir, P.; Wright, F.V.; McCrindle, B.; et al. Validation of the Actiheart activity monitor for measurement of activity energy expenditure in children and adolescents with chronic disease. *Eur. J. Clin. Nutr.* **2010**, *64*, 1494–1500. [CrossRef]
5. Collins, P.W.; Hamilton, M.; Dunstan, F.D.; Maguire, S.; Nuttall, D.E.; Liesner, R.; Thomas, A.E.; Hanley, J.; Chalmers, E.; Blanchette, V.; et al. Patterns of bruising in preschool children with inherited bleeding disorders: A longitudinal study. *Arch. Dis. Child.* **2017**, *102*, 1110–1117. [CrossRef]
6. Stephensen, D.; Drechsler, W.I.; Scott, O.M. Outcome measures monitoring physical function in children with haemophilia: A systematic review. *Haemophilia* **2014**, *20*, 306–321. [CrossRef]
7. Von Mackensen, S. Quality of life and sports activities in patients with haemophilia. *Haemophilia* **2007**, *13*, 38–43. [CrossRef]
8. Iorio, A.; Fabbriciani, G.; Marcucci, M.; Brozzetti, M.; Filipponi, P. Bone mineral density in haemophilia patients: A meta-analysis. *Thromb. Haemost.* **2010**, *103*, 596–603. [CrossRef]
9. Khair, K.; Littley, A.; Will, A.; von Mackensen, S. The impact of sport on children with haemophilia. *Haemophilia* **2012**, *18*, 898–905. [CrossRef]
10. Nixon, P.A.; Orenstein, D.M.; Kelsey, S.F. Habitual physical activity in children and adolescents with cystic fibrosis. *Med. Sci. Sports Exerc.* **2001**, *33*, 30–35. [CrossRef]
11. Gomis, M.; Querol, F.; Gallach, J.E.; González, L.M.; Aznar, J.A. Exercise and sport in the treatment of haemophilic patients: A systematic review. *Haemophilia* **2009**, *15*, 43–54. [CrossRef]
12. Hoefnagels, J.W.; Versloot, O.; Schrijvers, L.H.; van der Net, J.; Leebeek, F.W.G.; Gouw, S.C.; Fischer, K. Sports participation is not associated with adherence to prophylaxis in Dutch patients with haemophilia. *Haemophilia* **2021**. [CrossRef]
13. Cuesta-Barriuso, R.; Torres-Ortuño, A.; Pérez-Alenda, S.; Carrasco, J.J.; Querol, F.; Nieto-Munuera, J. Sporting activities and quality of life in children with hemophilia: An observational study. *Pediatr. Phys. Ther.* **2016**, *28*, 453–459. [CrossRef]
14. Soucie, J.M.; Cianfrini, C.; Janco, R.L.; Kulkarni, R.; Hambleton, J.; Evatt, B.; Forsyth, A.; Geraghty, S.; Hoots, K.; Abshire, T.; et al. Joint range-of-motion limitations among young males with hemophilia: Prevalence and risk factors. *Blood* **2004**, *103*, 2467–2473. [CrossRef]
15. Philpott, J.; Houghton, K.; Luke, A. Physical activity recommendations for children with specific chronic health conditions: Juvenile idiopathic arthritis, hemophilia, asthma and cystic fibrosis Society, Canadian Paediatric Living, Healthy Active Committee, Medicine Sport, Paediatric. *Paediatr. Child Health* **2010**, *15*, 213–218. [CrossRef]
16. Longmuir, P.E.; Yap, L.A.; Bravo, C.; Lee, S.L.; Brandão, L.R. Childhood physical activity body contact risk: Feasibility of a novel technique for objective measurements of impact speed, frequency, and intentionality. *Haemophilia* **2016**, *22*, 126–133. [CrossRef]
17. Buzzard, B.M. Sports and Hemophilia-Antagonist or Protagonist. *Clin. Orthop. Relat. Res.* **1996**, *328*, 25–30. [CrossRef]
18. Wang, M.; Alvarez-Román, M.T.; Chowdary, P.; Quon, D.V.; Schafer, K. Physical activity in individuals with haemophilia and experience with recombinant factor VIII Fc fusion protein and recombinant factor IX Fc fusion protein for the treatment of active patients: A literature review and case reports. *Blood Coagul. Fibrinolysis* **2016**, *27*, 737–744. [CrossRef]
19. McLain, L.G.; Heldrich, F.T. Hemophilia and Sports. *Phys. Sportsmed.* **1990**, *18*, 73–80. [CrossRef]
20. Howell, C.; Scott, K.; Patel, D.R. Sports participation recommendations for patients with bleeding disorders. *Transl. Pediatr.* **2017**, *6*, 174–180. [CrossRef]
21. Ross, C.; Goldenberg, N.A.; Hund, D.; Manco-Johnson, M.J. Athletic participation in severe hemophilia: Bleeding and joint outcomes in children on prophylaxis. *Pediatrics* **2009**, *124*, 1267–1272. [CrossRef]
22. Manco-Johnson, M.J. Collision sports and risk of bleeding in children with hemophilia. *JAMA* **2012**, *308*, 1480–1481. [CrossRef]
23. Keller, K. American Academy of Pediatrics. Trampolines at Home, School, and Recreational Centers. *Encycl. Obes.* **2014**, *2021*. [CrossRef]
24. LeBlanc, C.M.A.; Purcell, L. Policy statement—Boxing participation by children and adolescents. *Pediatrics* **2011**, *128*, 617–623. [CrossRef]
25. Halstead, M.E.; Walter, K.D.; Moffatt, K. Sport-related concussion in children and adolescents. *Pediatrics* **2018**, *142*. [CrossRef]
26. Khair, K.; Gibson, F.; Meerabeau, L. The benefits of prophylaxis: Views of adolescents with severe haemophilia. *Haemophilia* **2012**, *18*, e286–e289. [CrossRef]

27. Kondo, Y.; Shida, Y.; Ishikawa, T.; Yada, K.; Takeyama, M.; Shima, M.; Nogami, K. A case of moderate haemophilia A with inhibitor, carrying the p.R1800H mutation, complicated with juvenile idiopathic arthritis. *Haemophilia* **2019**, *25*, e51–e54. [CrossRef]
28. Mercan, A.; Sarper, N.; Inanır, M.; Mercan, H.I.; Zengin, E.; Kılıç, S.C.; Gökalp, A.S. Hemophilia-specific quality of life index (Haemo-QoL and Haem-A-QoL Questionnaires) of children and adults: Result of a single center from Turkey. *Pediatr. Hematol. Oncol.* **2010**, *27*, 449–461. [CrossRef]
29. Mannucci, P.M.; Canciani, M.T.; Rota, L.; Donovan, B.S. Response of Factor VIII/von Willebrand Factor to DDAVP in Healthy Subjects and Patients with Haemophilia A and von Willebrand's Disease. *Br. J. Haematol.* **1981**, *47*, 283–293. [CrossRef]
30. Oldenburg, J.; Pavlova, A. Genetic risk factors for inhibitors to factors VIII and IX. *Haemophilia* **2006**, *12*, 15–22. [CrossRef]
31. Astermark, J.; Altisent, C.; Batorova, A.; Diniz, M.J.; Gringeri, A.; Holme, P.A.; Karafoulidou, A.; Lopez-Fernández, M.F.; Reipert, B.M.; Rocino, A.; et al. Non-genetic risk factors and the development of inhibitors in haemophilia: A comprehensive review and consensus report. *Haemophilia* **2010**, *16*, 747–766. [CrossRef]
32. Broderick, C.R.; Herbert, R.D.; Latimer, J.; Barnes, C.; Curtin, J.A.; Mathieu, E.; Monagle, P.; Brown, S.A. Association between physical activity and risk of bleeding in children with hemophilia. *JAMA* **2012**, *308*, 1452–1459. [CrossRef]
33. Coleman, N.; Nemeth, B.A.; Leblanc, C.M.A. Increasing Wellness through Physical Activity in Children with Chronic Disease and Disability. *Curr. Sports Med. Rep.* **2018**, *17*, 425–432. [CrossRef]
34. Mulder, K.; Cassis, F.; Seuser, D.R.A.; Narayan, P.; Dalzell, R.; Poulsen, W. Risks and benefits of sports and fitness activities for people with haemophilia. *Haemophilia* **2004**, *10*, 161–163. [CrossRef]
35. Valizadeh, L.; Hosseini, F.A.; Zamanzadeh, V.; Heidarnezhad, F.; Jasemi, M.; Lankarani, K.B. Practice of Iranian adolescents with hemophilia in prevention of complications of hemophilia. *Indian J. Palliat. Care* **2015**, *21*, 328–337. [CrossRef]
36. Keeling, D.; Tait, C.; Makris, M. Guideline on the selection and use of therapeutic products to treat haemophilia and other hereditary bleeding disorders. *Haemophilia* **2008**, *14*, 671–684. [CrossRef]
37. Broderick, C.R.; Herbert, R.D.; Latimer, J.; van Doorn, N. Patterns of physical activity in children with haemophilia. *Haemophilia* **2013**, *19*, 59–64. [CrossRef]
38. Bertamino, M.; Riccardi, F.; Banov, L.; Svahn, J.; Molinari, A. Hemophilia Care in the Pediatric Age. *J. Clin. Med.* **2017**, *6*, 54. [CrossRef]
39. Williams, V.K.; Antoniou, G.; Jackson, A.; Atkins, A. Parents' perception of quality of life in their sons with haemophilia. *J. Paediatr. Child Health* **2016**, *52*, 1095–1098. [CrossRef]
40. Mcgee, S.; Raffini, L.; Witmer, C. Organized sports participation and the association with injury in paediatric patients with haemophilia. *Haemophilia* **2015**, *21*, 538–542. [CrossRef]
41. Witmer, C.M. How I approach managing student athletes at risk for bleeding. *Pediatr. Blood Cancer* **2019**, *66*, e27523. [CrossRef] [PubMed]
42. Philpott, J.F.; Houghton, K.; Luke, A. Physical activity recommendations for children with specific chronic health conditions: Juvenile idiopathic arthritis, Hemophilia, Asthma, and Cystic fibrosis. *Clin. J. Sport Med.* **2010**, *20*, 167–172. [CrossRef] [PubMed]
43. Seuser, A.; Böhm, P.; Wermes, C. Early orthopaedic challenges in haemophilia patients and therapeutic approach. *Thromb. Res.* **2014**, *134*, S61–S67. [CrossRef] [PubMed]
44. Groen, W.G.; Takken, T.; Van Der Net, J.; Helders, P.J.M.; Fischer, K. Habitual physical activity in Dutch children and adolescents with haemophilia. *Haemophilia* **2011**, *17*, 906–912. [CrossRef]
45. Simmons, G.M.; Frick, N.; Wang, A.; Miller, M.E.; Fragueiro, D. Identifying information needs among children and teens living with haemophilia. *Haemophilia* **2014**, *20*, 1–8. [CrossRef]
46. Kuijlaars, I.A.R.; van der Net, J.; Schutgens, R.E.G.; Fischer, K. The Paediatric Haemophilia Activities List (pedHAL) in routine assessment: Changes over time, child-parent agreement and informative domains. *Haemophilia* **2019**, *25*, 953–959. [CrossRef]
47. Sondermann, J.; Herbsleb, M.; Stanek, F.D.; Gabriel, H.; Kentouche, K. Health promotion for young patients with haemophilia: Counselling, adjuvant exercise therapy and school sports. *Hamostaseologie* **2017**, *37*, 107–116. [CrossRef]
48. Taha, M.Y.; Hassan, M.K. Health-related quality of life in children and adolescents with hemophilia in Basra, Southern Iraq. *J. Pediatr. Hematol. Oncol.* **2014**, *36*, 179–184. [CrossRef]
49. Kumar, R.; Bouskill, V.; Schneiderman, J.E.; Pluthero, F.G.; Kahr, W.H.A.; Craik, A.; Clark, D.; Whitney, K.; Zhang, C.; Rand, M.L.; et al. Impact of aerobic exercise on haemostatic indices in paediatric patients with haemophilia: Results from a prospective cohort study. *Thromb. Haemost.* **2016**, *115*, 1120–1128. [CrossRef]
50. Timmer, M.A.; Gouw, S.C.; Feldman, B.M.; Zwagemaker, A.; De Kleijn, P.; Pisters, M.F.; Schutgens, R.E.G.; Blanchette, V.; Srivastava, A.; David, J.A.; et al. Measuring activities and participation in persons with haemophilia: A systematic review of commonly used instruments. *Haemophilia* **2018**, *24*, e33–e49. [CrossRef]
51. Mannucci, P.M.; Direction, S. Treatment of haemophilia: Building on strength in the third millennium. *Haemophilia* **2012**, *17*, 1–24.
52. Wagner, B.; Seuser, A.; Krüger, S.; Herzig, M.L.; Hilberg, T.; Ay, C.; Hasenöhrl, T.; Crevenna, R. Establishing an online physical exercise program for people with hemophilia. *Wien. Klin. Wochenschr.* **2019**, *131*, 558–566. [CrossRef] [PubMed]
53. Wu, R.; Luke, K.-H.; Poon, M.-C.; Wu, X.; Zhang, N.; Zhao, L.; Su, Y.; Zhang, J. Low dose secondary prophylaxis reduces joint bleeding in severe and moderate haemophilic children: A pilot study in China. *Haemophilia* **2011**, *17*, 70–74. [CrossRef] [PubMed]
54. Broderick, C.R.; Herbert, R.D.; Latimer, J.; Curtin, J.A. Fitness and quality of life in children with haemophilia. *Haemophilia* **2010**, *16*, 118–123. [CrossRef]

55. Limperg, P.F.; Joosten, M.M.H.; Fijnvandraat, K.; Peters, M.; Grootenhuis, M.A.; Haverman, L. Male gender, school attendance and sports participation are positively associated with health-related quality of life in children and adolescents with congenital bleeding disorders. *Haemophilia* **2018**, *24*, 395–404. [CrossRef]
56. Khair, K.; Holland, M.; Bladen, M.; Griffioen, A.; McLaughlin, P.; Von Mackensen, S. Study of physical function in adolescents with haemophilia: The SO-FIT study. *Haemophilia* **2017**, *23*, 918–925. [CrossRef] [PubMed]
57. Von Mackensen, S.; Harrington, C.; Tuddenham, E.; Littley, A.; Will, A.; Fareh, M.; Hay, C.R.; Khair, K. The impact of sport on health status, psychological well-being and physical performance of adults with haemophilia. *Haemophilia* **2016**, *22*, 521–530. [CrossRef]

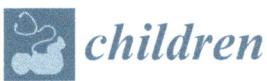

Communication

Interobserver Reliability of Pirani and Dimeglio Scores in the Clinical Evaluation of Idiopathic Congenital Clubfoot

Vito Pavone *, Andrea Vescio *, Annalisa Culmone, Alessia Caldaci, Piermario La Rosa, Luciano Costarella and Gianluca Testa

Department of General Surgery and Medical Surgical Specialties, Section of Orthopaedics and Traumatology, University Hospital Policlinico "Rodolico-San Marco", University of Catania, 95123 Catania, Italy; annalisa.culmone@libero.it (A.C.); alessia.c.92@hotmail.it (A.C.); larosapiermario@gmail.com (P.L.R.); lcostarella@yahoo.it (L.C.); gianpavel@hotmail.com (G.T.)
* Correspondence: vitopavone@hotmail.com (V.P.); andreavescio88@gmail.com (A.V.)

Abstract: Background: Dimeglio (DimS) and Pirani (PirS) scores are the most common scores used in congenital talipes equinovarus (CTEV) clinical practice. The aim of this study was to evaluate the interobserver reliability of these scores and how clinical practice can influence the clinical outcome of clubfoot through the DimS and Pirs. Methods: Fifty-four feet were assessed by six trained independent observers through the DimS and PirS: three consultants (OS), and three residents (RS) divided into three pediatric orthopaedic surgeons (PeO) and three non-pediatric orthopaedic surgeons (NPeO). Results: The PirS and DimS Scores were strongly correlated. In the same way, OS and RS, PirS, and DimS scores were strongly correlated, and the interobserver reliability ranked "good" in the comparison between PeO and NPeO. In fully trained paediatric orthopaedic surgeons, an "excellent" interobserver reliability was found but was only "good" in the NPeO cohort. Conclusions: In conclusion, after careful preparation, at least six months of observation of children with CTEV, PirS and DimS proved to be valid in terms of clinical evaluation. However, more experience with CTEV leads to a better clinical evaluation.

Keywords: clubfoot; Pirani score; Dimeglio score; interobserver reliability; congenital talipes equinovarus

1. Introduction

Congenital talipes equinovarus (CTEV) is one of the most common congenital pediatric orthopaedic deformities, characterised by dorsal hyperflexion of the foot, varus hindfoot, adduction of the hindfoot compared to the forefoot, and increased plantar arch [1]. Clinical manifestations might depend on aetiology [1], severity, and clinical course [2,3].

To achieve uniform clinical assessments and to provide the number of casts prediction or the tenotomy need, several authors have proposed different evaluation scores. In the early 1980s, Ponseti and Smoley [4] described a clinical manifestation-based tool aimed to assess the CTEVs and provide prognosis information. Their classification system was based on ankle dorsiflexion, heel varus, forefoot supination, and tibial torsion [2]. In 1983, Harrold and Walker [5] designated a deformity correction-based classification. Subsequently, Catterall et al. described a new score [6]; the questionnaire considered four patterns depending on the evolution of the deformity. Goldner et al. [7] reported a detailed score system that grades feet from 1 to 100. The authors provided a valid tool in the recurrent deformity prediction despite the significant variation in learning curve and reliability. Moreover, 18 out of 100 points are determined radiographically. In 1995, Dimeglio et al. [8] (DimS) designed a questionnaire with the purpose of analysing the severity to obtain reference points, assess the efficacy of orthopaedic treatment, and analyse the operative results objectively. In a retrospective classification systems comparison, Wainwright et al. [2] individuated DimS as a complex and effective score with the best agreement. In the same year, Pirani et al. (PirS) [9] included most of the elements of Catterall's method, but it is simpler to use for statistical comparisons [10].

At present, the most used evaluation scores are DimS and PirS [11–13], and these play a preponderant role in the clubfoot diagnosis and the treatment with the Ponseti.

The aim of our study is to evaluate the interobserver reliability of PirS and DimS scores and to evaluate how clinical practice can influence the proper severity of CTEV assessment. It was hypothesised that PirS and DimS are valid tools in clubfoot assessment with good interobserver reliability. Moreover, more skilled surgeons could report a superior observers' agreement.

2. Materials and Methods

2.1. General Information

Between 1st September 2019 and 26th April 2020, a review of all infants younger than 6 months of age at the first cast who underwent the Ponseti method for idiopathic CTEV at our institution was carried out. All patients were admitted through the pediatric orthopaedic ambulatory with the following demographic and clinical data captured: gender, age at treatment, the involved side, and presence or absence of associated syndromes or deformities. In addition, numbers of casts and age at the surgery were collected from the medical records. The inclusion criteria were as follows: (1) confirmed diagnosis of CTEV; (2) bilateral CTEV; (3) chronological age under six months; (4) treatment with Ponseti method; and (5) complete adherence to casting program.

The exclusion criteria were neurologic and syndromic clubfeet and postural deformities; patients older than six months of age; initial treatment or previous surgery in other institutions; follow-up less than six months; and incomplete adherence to the casting program.

All cases were treated by the same paediatric orthopaedic team with experience in clubfoot treatment using the Ponseti method.

2.2. Clinical Severity Assessments

2.2.1. Dimeglio Score (DimS)

Four clinical signs (varus, equinus, midfoot adduction, and derotation) of the calcaneo-forefoot block are evaluated in DimS. A points system based on reducibility on the relative plane, from zero to four, can be assigned to each item. Additional points were added for pre-operative deep posterior crease (1 point), deep medial crease (1 point), cavus (1 point), and muscle abnormalities (1 point). The final score can range from zero to 20 points, where a higher score indicates a more severe deformity. The severity of the deformity is then graded I–IV based on this scoring [8].

2.2.2. Pirani Score (PirS)

PirS assesses six clinical signs characterising clubfoot, three items for the midfoot, and three for the hindfoot: medial crease (MC-Pir), lateral part of the head of the talus, the curvature of the lateral border, posterior crease, empty heel, and rigid equinus. Each of the six items are scored on a three-point scale (0 = none, 0.5 = moderate, 1 = severe abnormality). The total score ranges from 0 to 6 based on the severity of the deformity of the examined foot [10].

2.2.3. Evaluation Contributors

All CTEV children included in the study were independently examined and assessed by three different orthopaedic surgeons (OS) and three resident doctors (RD) involved in pediatric orthopaedic care. All evaluators had previous experience of at least six months with these scoring systems. Three assessors, two OS and an RD, had a complete, full-trained program in pediatric orthopaedics (PeO) and treated more than 20 CTEV patients in the previous two years. An OS had a complete, full-trained program in foot and ankle diseases, while two RDs had at least one year of experience in the clubfoot treatment (NPeO). All the observers underwent 1 h of theoretical CTEV clinical manifestation and scoring system training before the CTEVs assessment.

2.3. Primary Outcome Measurement

To assess the interobserver reliability of PirS and DimS at different severities of the deformity, the intra-class correlation coefficients (ICC) statistic test was performed.

2.4. Secondary Outcome Measurement

To assess the importance of the experience, two cohort comparisons were performed. In the first, we compared the OS and RS; in the second, we compared the PeO and NPeO results.

2.5. Statistical Analysis

Continuous data are presented as means and standard deviations, as appropriate. The ICC (two-way random effects model, single-measure reliability) was performed to evaluate the observers' agreement. According to the Koo and Li [14] guideline, agreement below 0.50 was considered as "poor"; between 0.50 and 0.74 as "moderate"; between 0.75 and 0.89 as "good"; and above 0.90 as "excellent". The Pearson correlation coefficient (PCC) was utilised to assess the correlation between the scores. The PCC between 0.0 and 0.09 was considered "negligible"; between 0.1 and 0.39 as "weak"; between 0.40 and 0.69 as "moderate"; between 0.7 and 0.89 as "strong", and between 0.9 and 1.0 as "very strong" [15]. A Bland and Altman plot was produced to analyse the differences between the cohorts measurements. The limits of agreement (LOA) were calculated as the mean difference $\pm$ 1.96 standard deviations (SD) [16].

3. Results

Twenty-seven (18 females and 9 males) patients were considered eligible and included in the study. A total of 54 feet were assessed by six independent observers. The mean age at the first cast was 22 ± 11 days. The mean PirS at the first cast was 4.9 ± 1.0, while the mean DimS was 3.2 ± 0.9. The median of cast numbers was 6 ± 2. In all cases, the Achilles tenotomy was performed.

3.1. PirS and DimS Interobserver Reliability

According to the Koo and Li guideline [14], the PirS ICC between the six observers was 0.80 (95% confidence interval 0.69–0.86), classified as "good". The DimS ICC observed was 0.81 (95% confidence interval 0.74–0.87) and considered as "good". A "strong" correlation between the scores was found according to Schober et al. classification (PCC = 0.89 ($p < 0.001$)).

3.2. OS and RS Scores' Interobserver Reliability

The PirS ICC between the OS cohort was 0.80 (95% confidence interval 0.70–0.86), while RS PirS ICC was 0.82 (95% confidence interval 0.74–0.89), and both were considered "good" (Figure 1).

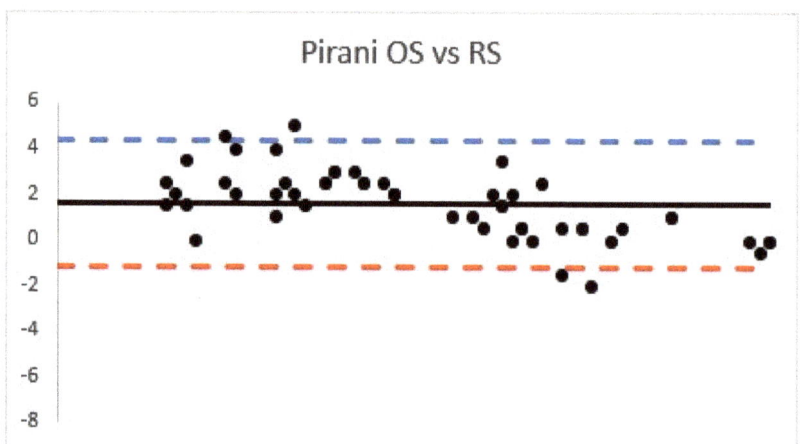

Figure 1. Bland Altman plots according to OS and RS Pirani score.

The DimS ICC observed was classified as "good" for both the cohorts (OS ICC = 0.78 (95% confidence interval 0.68–0.86); RS ICC = 0.80 (95% confidence interval 0.70–0.87)) (Figure 2).

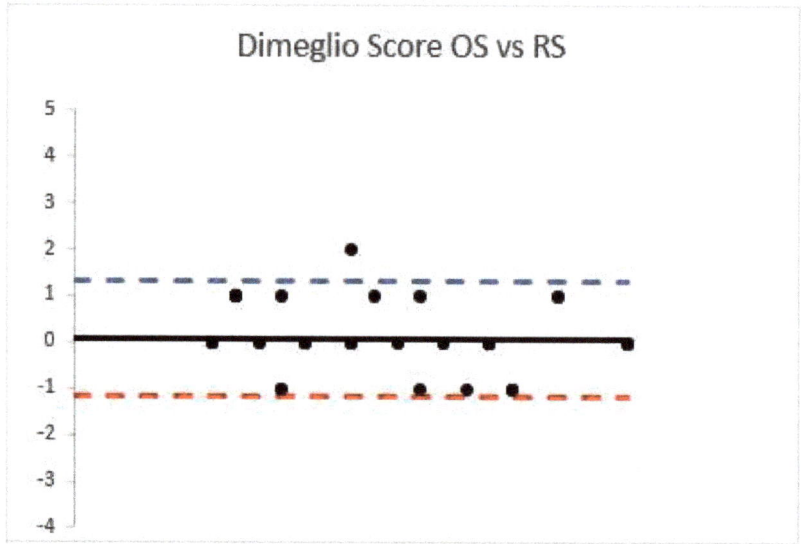

Figure 2. Bland Altman plots according to OS and RS Dimeglio score.

A strong correlation was observed according the PirS PCC (0.87 ($p < 0.001$)) and DimS PCC was 0.85 ($p < 0.001$) and classified as "strong".

3.3. PeO and NPeO Scores' Interobserver Reliability

The PirS ICC between the PeO cohort was 0.95 (95% confidence interval, 0.92–0.97) and considered "excellent", while NPeO PirS ICC was 0.76 (95% confidence interval, 0.66–0.84) and classified as "good" (Figure 3).

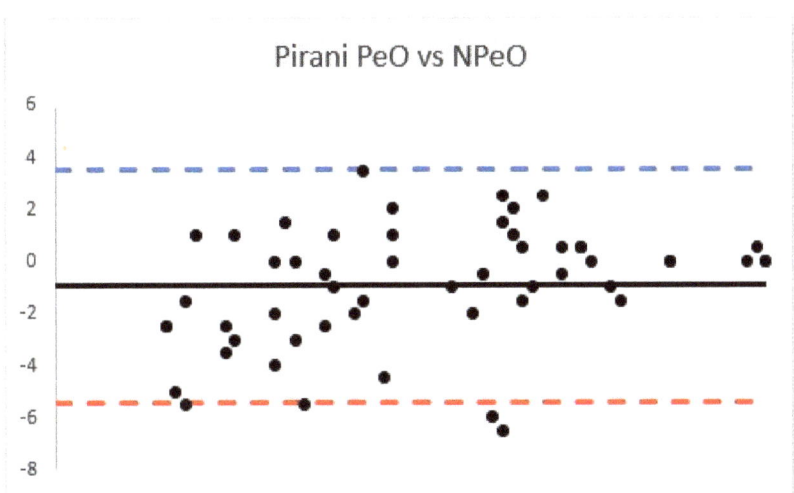

Figure 3. Bland Atman plots according to OS and RS Pirani score.

The DimS ICC observed was classified as "excellent" for PeO group (ICC = 0.91 (95% confidence interval 0.87–0.95), while NPeO DimS ICC was 0.80 (95% confidence interval 0.70–0.87) and considered "good" (Figure 4).

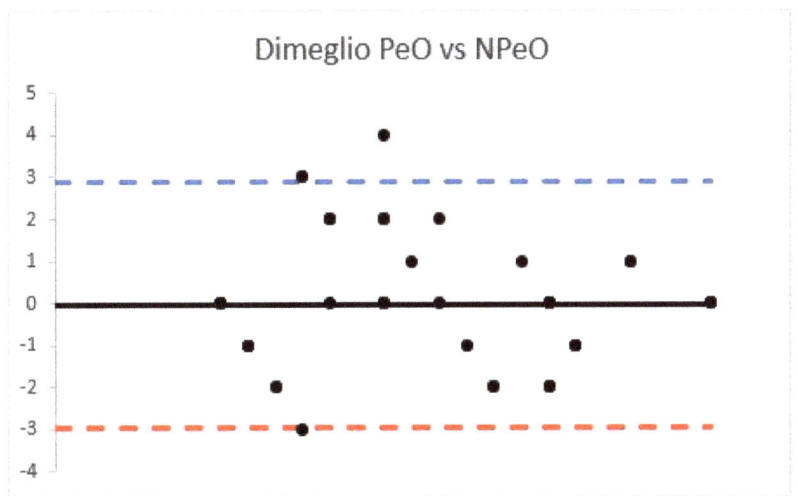

Figure 4. Bland Altman plots according to OS and RS Dimeglio score.

Considering the PCC, strong correlations were found (PirS PCC = 0.76 ($p < 0.001$); DimS PCC = 0.75 ($p < 0.001$)).

4. Discussion

Based on our data, PirS and DimS are valid scores in the assessment of CTEV clinical manifestation. Both scores were strongly correlated and showed good interobserver reliability. Moreover, our findings highlighted that measurement training could play a crucial role in clinical evaluation. In pediatric orthopaedic disorders assessed by experienced observers, greater concordance in the assessment was found. Few studies have attempted to evaluate PirS and DimS score reliability assessments [2,8,10–12,17–23], and the comparison between the studies is challenging due to the different statistical evaluation methods used to calculate the agreement degree among the observers. Vasu et al. [24] analysed the prognostic efficacy of both scores and reported a high validity in terms of clinical and prognostic evaluation but not the superiority of a score. Mulker et al. [25] and Mejaby [13] confirmed the high prognostic validity of DimS and Pirs, respectively. Several authors [17,19,26] have verified the high reliability of the scores. According to previous findings, our data demonstrated a strong correlation between the scores and good interobserver reliability. Interestingly, in two studies [17], the authors investigated the inter-rater reliability of the total score and of the sub-parameters. Although both trials reported a high correlation of the total score of both questionnaires, a few sub-parameters were found with a low reliability degree. In particular, according to the kappa values (acceptable if >0.60), every sub-parameter highlighted poor reliability values except for the equinus and the curvature of the lateral border in PirS, 0.74 for the muscle abnormality in DimS [26].

Other authors [20,23] have investigated the role of experience in CTEV assessment but evaluated only a single questionnaire, the PirS. Shaheen et al. [20] analysed the interobserver reliability of PirS between a pediatric orthopaedic surgeon and a physiotherapy assistant and observed a moderate to substantial concordance [20]. Sharma et al. [23] enrolled orthopaedic surgeons, a resident doctor, and a nonmedical counsellor. The authors highlighted discreet-to-remarkable interobserver reliability of all the subcomponents. In our study, three orthopaedic surgeons and three orthopaedic residents were compared. In both cohorts, the interobserver reliability was "good". Moreover, a strong correlation was observed according to the PirS and DimS among the groups.

To our knowledge, this is the first study comparing pediatric orthopaedics trained surgeons and general orthopaedic surgeons. Despite good reliability and a strong correlation in the NPeO group, a remarkable degree of agreement was observed when comparing a full pediatric orthopaedic training and when more than 20 clubfeet were treated. It can be assumed the routine practice in clubfoot treatment can provide a more unbiased assessment than the simple training lessons.

The main limit of the study was the lack of individual sub-parameters evaluation. The study presents several strengths, including the number of observers.

5. Conclusions

In conclusion, PirS and DimS are valid scores for the clinical and prognostic evaluation of CTEV and have shown high interobserver reliability. After sufficient training, both scores are easily utilised in the CTEV clinical evaluation even in the less expert subject. On the other hand, orthopaedics with more practice in the treatment of clubfoot evidenced a superior concordance.

Author Contributions: Conceptualization, V.P.; methodology, A.V.; software, P.L.R.; validation, G.T.; formal analysis, A.C. (Alessia Caldaci); investigation, A.C. (Annalisa Culmone); resources, G.T.; data curation, A.V.; writing—original draft preparation, A.C. (Alessia Caldaci); writing—review and editing, G.T.; visualization, L.C.; supervision, V.P.; project administration, V.P.; funding acquisition, V.P. All authors have read and agreed to the published version of the manuscript.

Funding: This research received no external funding.

Institutional Review Board Statement: Not applicable.

Informed Consent Statement: Not applicable.

Data Availability Statement: Not applicable.

Acknowledgments: All individuals included in this section have consented to the acknowledgement.

Conflicts of Interest: The authors declare no conflict of interest.

References

1. Pavone, V.; Chisari, E.; Vescio, A.; Lucenti, L.; Sessa, G.; Testa, G. The etiology of idiopathic congenital talipes equinovarus: A systematic review. *J. Orthop. Surg. Res.* **2018**, *13*, 206. [CrossRef]
2. Wainwright, A.M.; Auld, T.; Benson, M.K.; Theologis, T.M. The classification of congenital talipes equinovarus. *J. Bone Joint Surg Br.* **2002**, *84*, 1020–1024. [CrossRef]
3. Pavone, V.; Bianca, S.; Grosso, G.; Pavone, P.; Mistretta, A.; Longo, M.R.; Marino, S.; Sessa, G. Congenital talipes equinovarus: An epidemiological study in Sicily. *Acta Orthop.* **2012**, *83*, 294–298. [CrossRef]
4. Ponseti, I.V.; Smoley, E.N. Congenital club foot: The results of treatment. *J. Bone Joint Surg. Am.* **1963**, *45*, 261–344. [CrossRef]
5. Harrold, A.J.; Walker, C.J. Treatment and prognosis in congenital club foot. *J. Bone Joint Surg Br.* **1983**, *65*, 8–11. [CrossRef]
6. Catterall, A. A method of assessment of the clubfoot deformity. *Clin. Orthop. Relat. Res.* **1991**, *264*, 48–53. [CrossRef]
7. Goldner, J.; Fitch, R. Classification and evaluation of congenital talipes equinovarus. In *The Clubfoot*; Simons, G.W., Ed.; Springer: New York, NY, USA, 1993; pp. 120–139.
8. Diméglio, A.; Bensahel, H.; Souchet, P.; Mazeau, P.; Bonnet, F. Classification of clubfoot. *J. Pediatr. Orthop. B* **1995**, *4*, 129–136. [CrossRef] [PubMed]
9. Pirani, S.; Outerbridge, H.; Moran, M.; Sawatsky, B. A method of evaluating the virgin clubfoot with substantial inter-observer reliability. Available online: https://ci.nii.ac.jp/naid/10027866447/ (accessed on 20 June 2021).
10. Flynn, J.M.; Donohoe, M.; Mackenzie, W.G. An independent assessment of two clubfoot-classification systems. *J. Pediatr. Orthop.* **1998**, *18*, 323–327. [CrossRef] [PubMed]
11. Harvey, N.J.; Mudge, A.J.; Daley, D.T.; Sims, S.K.; Adams, R.D. Inter-rater reliability of physiotherapists using the Pirani scoring system for clubfoot: Comparison with a modified five-point scale. *J. Pediatr. Orthop. B* **2014**, *23*, 493–500. [CrossRef] [PubMed]
12. Cosma, D.; Vasilescu, D.E. A Clinical Evaluation of the Pirani and Dimeglio Idiopathic Clubfoot Classifications. *J. Foot Ankle Surg.* **2015**, *54*, 582–585. [CrossRef]
13. Mejabi, J.O.; Esan, O.; Adegbehingbe, O.O.; Orimolade, E.A.; Asuquo, J.; Badmus, H.D.; Anipole, A. The Pirani Scoring System is Effective in Assessing Severity and Monitoring Treatment of Clubfeet in Children. *Br. J. Med. Med. Res.* **2016**, *17*, 1–9. [CrossRef]
14. Koo, T.K.; Li, M.Y. A Guideline of Selecting and Reporting Intraclass Correlation Coefficients for Reliability Research. *J. Chiropr. Med.* **2016**, *15*, 155–163. [CrossRef]
15. Schober, P.; Boer, C.; Schwarte, L.A. Correlation Coefficients: Appropriate Use and Interpretation. *Anesth. Analg.* **2018**, *126*, 1763–1768. [CrossRef]
16. Altman, D.G.; Bland, J.M. Assessing Agreement between Methods of Measurement. *Clin. Chem.* **2017**, *63*, 1653–1654. [CrossRef] [PubMed]
17. Lampasi, M.; Abati, C.N.; Bettuzzi, C.; Stilli, S.; Trisolino, G. Comparison of Dimeglio and Pirani score in predicting number of casts and need for tenotomy in clubfoot correction using the Ponseti method. *Int. Orthop.* **2018**, *42*, 2429–2436. [CrossRef] [PubMed]
18. Pirani, S.; Hodges, D.; Sekeramyi, F. A reliable and valid method of assessing the amount of deformity in the congenital clubfoot deformity. *J. Bone Joint Surg. Br.* **2008**, *90*, 53.
19. Fan, H.; Liu, Y.; Zhao, L.; Chu, C.; An, Y.; Wang, T.; Li, W. The Correlation of Pirani and Dimeglio Scoring Systems for Ponseti Management at Different Levels of Deformity Severity. *Sci. Rep.* **2017**, *7*, 14578. [CrossRef]
20. Shaheen, S.; Jaiballa, H.; Pirani, S. Interobserver reliability in Pirani clubfoot severity scoring between a paediatric orthopaedic surgeon and a physiotherapy assistant. *J. Pediatr. Orthop. B* **2012**, *21*, 366–368. [CrossRef]
21. Jillani, S.A.; Aslam, M.Z.; Chinoy, M.A.; Khan, M.A.; Saleem, A.; Ahmed, S.K. A comparison between orthopedic surgeon and allied health worker in Pirani score. *J. Pak. Med. Assoc.* **2014**, *64*, 127–130.
22. Jain, S.; Ajmera, A.; Solanki, M.; Verma, A. Interobserver variability in Pirani clubfoot severity scoring system between the orthopedic surgeons. *Indian, J. Orthop.* **2017**, *51*, 81–85. [CrossRef]
23. Sharma, P.; Verma, R.; Gaur, S. Interobserver Reliability of Pirani Clubfoot Severity Scoring between an Orthopedic Surgeon, a Resident Doctor, and a Nonmedical Counsellor at a Clubfoot Clinic. *Indian J. Orthop.* **2018**, *52*, 645–650. [PubMed]
24. Chatterjee, V.D.; Gupta, V. Evaluation of idiopathic Clubfoot Deformity in Infants by Pirani or Dimeglio Score: Attempting to Clear the Confusion! *N. Indian J. Surg.* **2012**, *3*, 162.
25. Van Mulken, J.M.; Bulstra, S.K.; Hoefnagels, N.H. Evaluation of the treatment of clubfeet with the Dimeglio score. *J. Pediatr. Orthop.* **2001**, *21*, 642–647. [CrossRef]
26. Bettuzzi, C.; Abati, C.N.; Salvatori, G.; Zanardi, A.; Lampasi, M. Interobserver reliability of Dimeglio and Pirani score and their subcomponents in the evaluation of idiopathic clubfoot in a clinical setting: A need for improved scoring systems. *J. Child. Orthop.* **2019**, *13*, 478–485. [CrossRef] [PubMed]

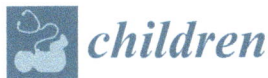

Case Report

A New Proximal Femur Reconstruction Technique after Bone Tumor Resection in a Very Small Patient: An Exemplificative Case

Carmine Zoccali [1], Silvia Careri [2,*], Dario Attala [3], Michela Florio [2], Giuseppe Maria Milano [4] and Marco Giordano [2]

[1] Oncological Orthopaedics Department, IRCCS—Regina Elena National Cancer Institute, Via Elio Chianesi 53, 00144 Rome, Italy; carmine.zoccali@ifo.gov.it
[2] Department of Orthopaedics and Traumatology, Bambino Gesù Children's Hospital, IRCCS, Piazza di Sant'Onofrio 4, 00165 Rome, Italy; michela.florio@opbg.net (M.F.); marco.giordano@opbg.net (M.G.)
[3] Muscular-Skeletal Tissue Bank–IRCCS–Regina Elena National Cancer Institute, Via Elio Chianesi 53, 00144 Rome, Italy; dario.attala@ifo.gov.it
[4] Department of Pediatric Hematology/Oncology and Stem Cell Transplantation, Bambino Gesù Children's Hospital, IRCCS, Piazza di Sant'Onofrio 4, 00165 Rome, Italy; giuseppemaria.milano@opbg.net
* Correspondence: silvia.careri@opbg.net; Tel.: +39-06-68592313

Abstract: For patients too young to be fitted with an expandable prosthesis, limb salvage surgery requires other strategies. The main problems are related to the impossibility of implanting an expandable prosthesis to the residual bone growth that is much too big in relation to the bone size, with the precocious implant loosening and/or the residual absence of bone growth, as well as the problem of limb length and shape difference. In this paper, we report a possible reconstruction solution using a composite prosthesis for an Ewing's sarcoma of the proximal femur in an infant patient. After resection, a femoral stem was cemented into the distal third of a homoplastic humerus; a carbon fiber plate was used to stabilize the bone/homograft interface. At the one-year follow-up, the patient was free of disease and able to walk with only a slight limp. This case report describes a possible solution for very small patients. An adult humerus is of the right size to replace a child's lower limb segments, and the distal humerus can be shaped, maintaining a cortex stiff enough to support a prosthesis. Very young patients might obtain a faster osteointegration of the graft than adults, due to their higher biological activity and, in this case, the diapasonal shape of the allograft might also have contributed to accelerated fusion. Moreover, the use of a graft to fit the prosthesis avoids loosening issues due to canal widening, hypothetically providing more growing time before system failure and revision surgery. However, although this technique is promising, further studies are necessary to confirm our findings and to verify if this procedure allows easier future prosthesis implantation.

Keywords: bone tumors; Ewing's sarcoma; infants; children; composite prosthesis

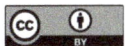

1. Background

Osteosarcoma and Ewing's sarcoma represent the most frequent malignant primary bone tumors occurring in skeletally immature patients. While osteosarcoma is more common in the second decade of life, predominantly affecting the knee, Ewing's sarcoma is also frequent in the first decade of life [1]. Treatments are multidisciplinary, and based on a combination of chemotherapy, radiotherapy and surgery [2]. Previously, amputation was considered the principal surgical treatment assuring a radical margin; however, improved chemotherapy schedules permit sparing the limb and increased survival [3,4].

Today, limb salvage surgery is considered the standard treatment for malignant tumors [5]. After bone tumor resection, the use of a megaprosthesis is considered the most common method of reconstruction [6]. This is true for adults and for fully grown patients; for growing patients, expandable prostheses can be a solution as long as the size of the bone segment permits the insertion of such a voluminous device [7,8].

In very small patients, in whom a prosthesis cannot be used, other strategies must be applied, and bone reconstruction becomes a challenging problem. Indeed, children have a different anatomy, so both resection and reconstruction are more difficult than in adults; moreover, modular prostheses are not commercially available in the required small sizes.

In fact, the main problems are related to bone growth, which could cause a precocious implant to mobilize due to the increasing bone diameter [9] and, obviously, the leg length discrepancy [10].

Possible solutions are as follows.

(1) Expandable prosthesis: this can be used only in older children where the residual bone is sufficiently long for a prosthesis with an elongation system to be inserted. Expandable prostheses are potentially able to compensate for the bone shortening after tumor resection, but results are poor due to loosening and breakage [9].

(2) Custom-made prosthesis: this is considered the most common treatment when modular prostheses are not available. Their use is very common in children. Custom-made prostheses can provoke aseptic loosening, and cause loss of bone stock, making revision surgery difficult and obtaining low functional results [11].

(3) Vascularized fibular flap: this technique was proposed by Manfrini et al., who replaced the femur by modeling the autogenous fibula, reproducing the femoral shape. The fibular epiphysis was used to imitate the femoral head [12]. The advantage of this technique is the potential growth of the fibula and its remodeling; nevertheless, it is a very difficult technique, and the success rate is quite low. Indeed, there are no case series in the literature.

(4) Extracorporeal irradiated autograft: this technique consists of reimplantation of the resected specimen after irradiation and soft tissue removal. It has the advantage of a perfect anatomical correspondence, although non-union is common [13]; moreover, it does not furnish complete information about histology and tumor necrosis after neoadjuvant chemotherapy. Although the hypothetical risk of local recurrence is present, it seems similar to that of other techniques which do not include the reimplantation of the specimen [14].

(5) Osteoarticular homograft: this is rarely used in isolation for the inferior limb, principally because it collapses under body weight and cannot articulate with the acetabulum, undergoing precocious resorption [15]. Moreover, these are not available for children, due to the absence of donors.

(6) Composite prosthesis (association of a joint prosthesis and a cemented homograft): this has the advantage of increasing the bone stock [16]; the prosthetic component should also guarantee a good articular motion. The corresponding homograft segment would be the best solution, but unfortunately, it is impossible to have child donors, so homografts from adult donors have to be adapted for young patients [10]. The homograft medullary canal is completely filled with cement in order to obtain higher resistance in weight-bearing.

In this paper we report a possible solution for reconstruction of the proximal femur in infant patients using a composite prosthesis; an exemplificative case is reported.

2. Case Report

A girl aged 2 years and 8 months presented with the presence of a mass, indicative of malignancy, in her right proximal femur, and complained of continuous pain and limping. An X-ray (Figure 1A), MRI, scintigraphy and a CT scan were performed, and showed an osteolytic lesion in the proximal and middle femur. The bone cortex was extensively disrupted, but the proximal and distal femur growth cartilage was free from disease.

The soft tissues mainly involved were the thigh anterior side muscles and, to a lesser extent, tissues in the posteromedial area, with the bone section globally embedded in the neoplasm; no metastases were detected, so a CT-trocar biopsy was performed. Histology revealed an Ewing's sarcoma, and the patient was administered neoadjuvant chemotherapy with vincristine, cyclophosphamide, and doxorubicin. The subsequent CT scan and MRI, performed for surgical planning, showed multiple osteolytic areas beginning 8 mm from the growth plate and extending for 80 mm from the femoral neck base (Figure 1B,C). The distal edge of the sarcoma was 63 mm from the distal physis.

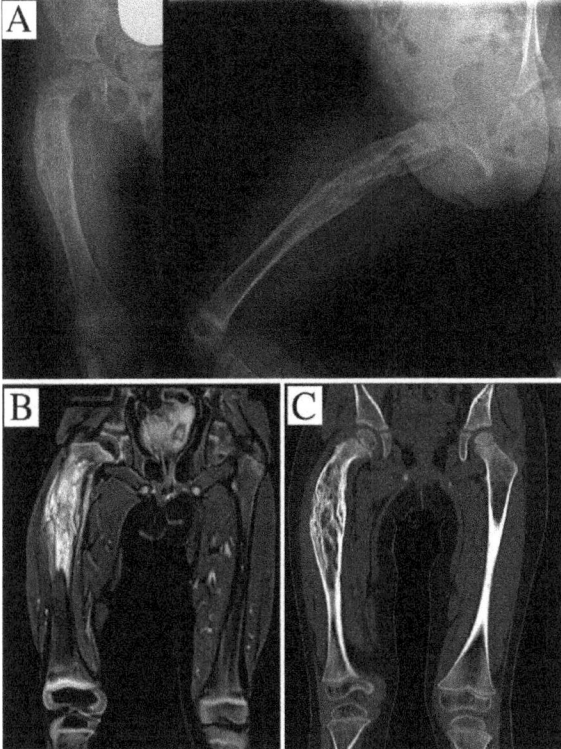

Figure 1. (**A**) an X-ray showing an osteolytic and apparently well-defined lesion of the proximal and middle third of the right femur; the segment is bent with onion-skin periosteal reaction; (**B**) STIR-weighted coronal-MRI reconstruction, evidencing permeative behavior and an intense edema. (**C**) CT scan showing the geographic osteolysis.

Surgery was performed in a specialized research hospital by a surgical team trained in musculoskeletal oncology, with more than 15 years' experience of exclusively performing musculoskeletal tumor operations, and an experienced pediatric orthopedic surgeon. With the patient in a left lateral position, a direct lateral approach was performed; the proximal and middle femur was isolated, maintaining a layer of muscles to guarantee a wide margin. A femoral osteotomy was performed at 14 cm from the greater trochanter, and the proximal femur was removed after capsulotomy and sectioning of the rounded ligament. A distal section of a homoplastic humerus was then used for reconstruction. The allograft was obtained from "Regione Lazio Muscular Skeletal Tissue Bank". It was stored frozen at −80 °C and not irradiated; bacteriologic and viral analyses were performed (with negative results), and before surgery, it was soaked in a Rifampicin antibiotic solution. The humeral medial epicondyle was removed; the olecranon fossa was drilled to access the medullary canal, and an adequate site for the implant was obtained using broaches (Figure 2A); then, a femoral stem prosthesis was cemented (Exeter DDH—Stryker, Kalamazoo, MI, USA) (Figure 2B). To increase the fusion, a diapason-shaped osteotomy was done in the distal extremity of the homograft and a cortical strut was placed and cemented inside to maintain the axis (Figure 2C).

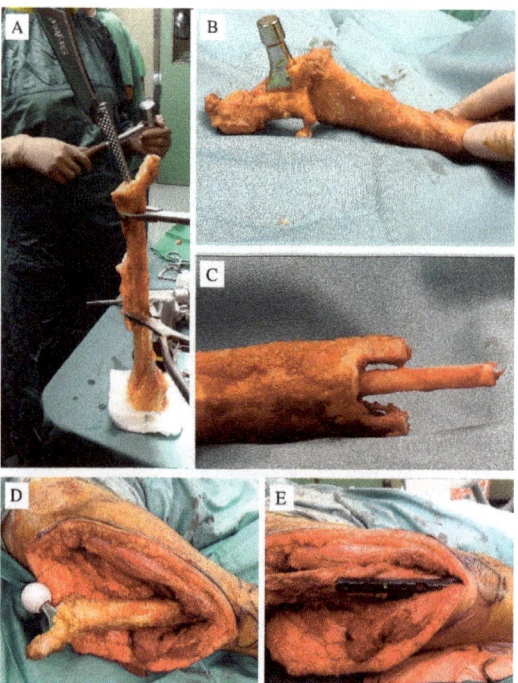

Figure 2. (**A**) The distal humerus after cutting of the medial epicondyle; the broaches were used to create a housing for the prosthesis; (**B**) the prosthesis cemented inside the canal; (**C**) the distal allograft was cut to a diapason shape to fit together with the patient's residual femur; a cortical strut was cemented in the allograft medullary canal to increase the primary stability when inserted in the residual distal femur; (**D**) a ceramic head of 28 mm was applied; (**E**) the carbon fiber plate and screws used to stabilize the contact area between the allograft and the patient's femur.

A 28 mm ceramic femoral head was applied, the construct was connected to the residual distal femur (Figure 2D) and distally stabilized with a carbon fiber plate and screws (CarboFix Orthopedics Ltd., carbon fiber plate, Herzeliya, Israel) (Figure 2E). A capsuloplasty was done to decrease the risk of dislocation, and the gluteus muscles were stitched to the residual epicondyle, mimicking the great trochanter to the residual soft tissue. A transfusion of 300 mL of erythrocytes was administered during surgery, due to intra-operative blood loss.

A single hip spica was applied for 40 days and was then replaced by a thigh–foot half-cast in order to begin hip movement while still protecting the graft-to-host junction. After 30 days, the cast was removed. The knee extension was complete, but the maximum flexion was limited to 30°. Physical therapy started, focusing on range of movement recovery of the knee, but still maintaining no weight-bearing for another 30 days. The postoperative histology evidenced the presence of a macroscopic viable tumor (necrosis inferior to 70%), grade I responder according to Picci et al. [17]; the surgical margin was wide, so adjuvant radiotherapy was not indicated. In the meantime, adjuvant chemotherapy with vincristine, cyclophosphamide and doxorubicin was administered.

At the one-year follow-up, the patient is apparently free of disease, and the allograft is completely osteointegrated (Figure 3). The young patient is able to walk with only a slight limp, as shown in Video S1 (link in Supplementary Materials). The right femur has been lengthened by 10 mm during surgery in order to reduce the leg length difference that will develop, and a 1-cm right shoe lift has been prescribed to obtain a temporary correction. Compared to the X-ray taken immediately after surgery, at the last follow-up, the distal femur had already grown 12 mm.

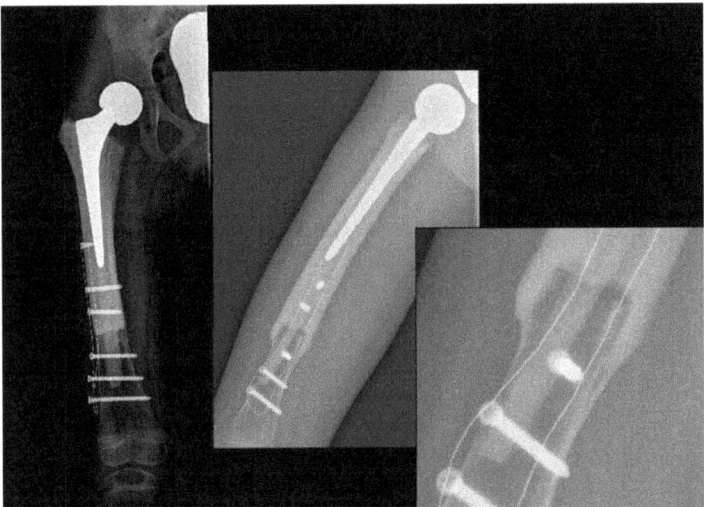

Figure 3. X-ray showing a stable fusion between the allograft and the femur.

The active hip range of motion (ROM) was flexion 80°, extension 10°, abduction 20°. The active knee joint ROM was: flexion 110° and extension 0°.

This study was conducted in accordance with the World Medical Association Declaration of Helsinki of 1975, as revised in 1983, and the patient's parents signed an informed consent form to allow the use of clinical data for research purposes and for publication. The local Ethics Committee approved the study (protocol number: 418/2021).

3. Discussion

Limb salvage surgery must be the goal to pursue when a wide resection of a tumor can be achieved. Thanks to sarcoma treatment improvement, the necessity for amputation has been reduced, but it maintains a fundamental role in certain cases [18]. At the same time, rotationplasty remains a viable option when limb-salvage is contraindicated [19], or if the distal femoral growth plate has to be sacrificed with consequent major limb length discrepancy [20]. The distal femoral growth plate of the patient was free from disease, and it was planned to spare it during surgery. As is known, distal femoral growth provides 70% of the bone length [21], thus, the use of the presented composite solution will allow the femur to grow to a near-normal length and width during the child's growing up. Moreover, preoperative examinations of our patient showed no involvement of the main vessels or nerves, no metastases, and adequate soft tissue coverage after surgery was expected. Taking these points into account, and clearly explaining to the patient's parents the expected necessity of further surgery and possible complications that could lead to amputation, the authors decided to pursue a limb-salvage solution.

The choice of a composite solution depended on different evaluations. A modular prosthesis of such a small size was not available. Moreover, there were concerns about two possible complications: first of all, the intramedullary stem perforation could compromise the distal femoral physis [22]. At the same time, due to the rapid growth of very young children, a rapid widening of the femoral canal was expected, with consequent loosening of the prosthesis.

The patient's fibula at the time of surgery had a 5 mm diameter. It is the authors' experience, also confirmed by Muscolo et al. [22], that younger children usually have good osteointegration, mostly when there is a good contact surface between the graft and the host bone. The possibility of a vascularized fibula graft was considered, but was rejected as the first choice because of the high failure rate.

The size of an adult femur is not suitable for reconstructing a child's femur, the diameter of the diaphysis and the femoral head being too wide. A skeletally mature humerus, however, has a size that is suitable for replacing segments of a child's femur or tibia.

The proximal humerus can also be used to reconstruct a child's proximal femur; indeed, it can support a small stem prosthesis and the residual capsule can be helpful for reattaching the gluteal muscles. However, the proximal epiphysis is quite big and may be much too bulky for very small patients, as in the presented case.

Furthermore, the anatomy of the distal humerus is more like that of the femur; the distal epiphysis can be shaped to reproduce the femur better than the proximal epiphysis. The cortex is stiff enough to support a prosthesis implant, and, if lateral ligaments are also available, they can be used to reattach the gluteal muscles.

After gaining access to the olecranon fossa and then to the medullary canal, the broaches can be easily manipulated to obtain a good fit to the distal humerus; a small endoprosthesis can be cemented in the allograft, obtaining good primary stability (Figure 2B).

In the presented case, no collateral ligament was present, so trans-bone stitches were used with a satisfactory result; this ensured quite normal walking. A good fusion was also reached; this could be due to the higher biological activity and remodeling in young bone but also to the diapasonal shape of the distal allograft, which increases the bone-to-bone contact area. In addition, the cortical strut, cemented in the allograft medullary canal and fitted in the patient's residual femoral canal, contributed to the primary stability and underwent remodeling.

Moreover, the carbon fiber plate may facilitate osteointegration because it stabilizes the segments in a more elastic manner than a titanium plate does; its radiolucency makes it possible to monitor graft fusion, and should ensure safer postoperative radiotherapy, due to the lower level of artifacts, if this is necessary [23,24]. The aim of overlapping the proximal plate edge and femoral stem is to prevent stress fractures of the graft by improving the load distribution.

Unfortunately, this surgery must be considered as just a temporary solution. With the growth of the patient, the increase in diameter of the acetabulum, and the onset of bone shortening, future operations will be unavoidable. When the dimension of the segments allows, a custom-made expandable prosthesis could be considered to decrease any difference in leg length.

Fortunately, the distal epiphyseal plate was spared, maintaining its growth potential. This could allow for a residual medullary canal large enough to house the prosthesis stem, and spare the epiphyseal plate as well; moreover, considering the good level of remodeling present at one year after surgery, it would be desirable that part of the homograft could be used to host the prosthesis stem, obviously after cement and cortical strut removal.

Furthermore, the greatest lengthening allowed by tight soft tissues (1 cm) was provided during surgery in order to delay successive elongation. Moreover, the use of a graft to fit the prosthesis avoided the problem of loosening due to canal widening, as may occur when a prosthesis is inserted in a growing bone. The use of the graft also allowed the preservation of bone stock.

Unfortunately, the proximal growth cartilage was too close to the tumor to be spared, but the choice of an endoprosthetic replacement allows the acetabular triradiate cartilage to continue to grow, also receiving the correct mechanical stress from a spherical femoral head.

Obviously, this technique also presents possible disadvantages related to the use of a homograft; indeed, its osteointegration is quite limited to the contact area (a few centimeters) so there is a resorption risk. Moreover, a frequent complication is a fracture that can barely heal. This is the most frequent cause of revision.

Reconstruction surgery in very young patients presents another important challenge to bear in mind: their post-operative and rehabilitation care. In the presented case, the hip had to be protected against possible dislocation as well as the graft-to-host junction, to allow graft fusion. It was therefore necessary to prevent the infant's movement and weight-bearing by using a cast.

The choice of postoperative rehabilitation steps could greatly influence the functional result; indeed, precocious mobilization and weight-bearing could increase the risk of dislocation, but prolonged immobilization could cause excessive muscular fibrosis and weakness.

Obviously, the correct equilibrium must be found, also taking into consideration the young patient's cooperability.

The present paper presents several limitations, particularly because it is a case report. However, our findings need to be confirmed in several further cases before they can be considered valid. In addition, more studies with long-term follow-up will be necessary to determine how to resolve problems related to patients' growth and future prosthesis implants.

Supplementary Materials: The following are available online at https://www.mdpi.com/article/10.3390/children8060442/s1: Video S1: A new proximal femur reconstruction technique after bone tumor resection in a very small patient: an exemplificative case.

Author Contributions: C.Z. participated in the treatment conception and performed surgery; he participated in the study design and interpretation of data and drafted part of the original manuscript; S.C. participated in the study design, acquisition and interpretation of data, she also drafted part of the original manuscript; M.F. performed surgery and participated in the acquisition of surgical data; D.A. and G.M.M. helped in the acquisition of clinical data and review of the manuscript; M.G. participated in the treatment conception and performed surgery, he also drafted part of the manuscript and participated in data interpretation. All authors have read and agreed to the published version of the manuscript.

Funding: This research received no external funding.

Institutional Review Board Statement: This case report involving patient data was in accordance with the ethical standards of the institutional and national research committees and with the 1964 Helsinki Declaration and its later amendments or comparable ethical standards.

Informed Consent Statement: The patient's parents gave written consent for clinical data management and for images to be used for research purposes and publication.

Conflicts of Interest: The authors declare no conflict of interest.

References

1. Granowetter, L.; Womer, R.; Devidas, M.; Krailo, M.; Wang, C.; Bernstein, M.; Marina, N.; Leavey, P.; Gebhardt, M.; Healey, J.; et al. Dose-intensified compared with standard chemotherapy for nonmetastatic ewing sarcoma family of tumors: A children's oncology group study. *J. Clin. Oncol.* **2009**, *27*, 2536–2541. [CrossRef]
2. Cirstoiu, C.; Cretu, B.; Serban, B.; Panti, Z.; Nica, M. Current review of surgical management options for extremity bone sarcomas. *EFORT Open Rev.* **2019**, *4*, 174–182. [CrossRef]
3. Hesla, A.C.; Papakonstantinou, A.; Tsagkozis, P. Current status of management and outcome for patients with ewing sarcoma. *Cancers* **2021**, *13*, 1202. [CrossRef] [PubMed]
4. Ferrari, S.; Palmerini, E. Adjuvant and neoadjuvant combination chemotherapy for osteogenic sarcoma. *Curr. Opin. Oncol.* **2007**, *19*, 341–346. [CrossRef] [PubMed]
5. Goryń, T.; Pieńkowski, A.; Szostakowski, B.; Zdzienicki, M.; Ługowska, I.; Rutkowski, P. Functional outcome of surgical treatment of adults with extremity osteosarcoma after megaprosthetic reconstruction-Single-center experience. *J. Orthop. Surg. Res.* **2019**, *14*. [CrossRef] [PubMed]
6. Pala, E.; Trovarelli, G.; Angelini, A.; Maraldi, M.; Berizzi, A.; Ruggieri, P. Megaprosthesis of the knee in tumor and revision surgery. *Acta Biomed.* **2017**, *88*, 129–138. [CrossRef]

7. Dukan, R.; Mascard, E.; Langlais, T.; Ouchrif, Y.; Glorion, C.; Pannier, S.; Bouthors, C. Long-term outcomes of non-invasive expandable endoprostheses for primary malignant tumors around the knee in skeletally-immature patients. *Arch. Orthop. Trauma Surg.* **2021**. [CrossRef] [PubMed]
8. Torner, F.; Segur, J.M.; Ullot, R.; Soldado, F.; Domenech, P.; DeSena, L.; Knorr, J. Non-invasive expandable prosthesis in musculoskeletal oncology paediatric patients for the distal and proximal femur. First results. *Int. Orthop.* **2016**, *40*, 1683–1688. [CrossRef]
9. Baumgart, R.; Lenze, U. Expandable endoprostheses in malignant bone tumors in children: Indications and limitations. *Recent Results Cancer Res.* **2009**, *179*, 59–73.
10. Campanacci, L.; Alì, N.; Casanova, J.M.P.S.; Kreshak, J.; Manfrini, M. Resurfaced allograft-prosthetic composite for proximal tibial reconstruction in children: Intermediate-term results of an original technique. *J. Bone Jt. Surg. Am. Vol.* **2015**, *97*, 241–250. [CrossRef]
11. Schindler, O.S.; Cannon, S.R.; Briggs, T.W.R.; Blunn, G.W. Stanmore custom-made extendible distal femoral replacements. Clinical experience in children with primary malignant bone tumours. *J. Bone Jt. Surg. Ser. B* **1997**, *79*, 927–937. [CrossRef]
12. Manfrini, M.; Innocenti, M.; Ceruso, M.; Mercuri, M. Original biological reconstruction of the hip in a 4-year-old girl. *Lancet* **2003**, *361*, 140–142. [CrossRef]
13. Oike, N.; Kawashima, H.; Ogose, A.; Hatano, H.; Ariizumi, T.; Kaidu, M.; Aoyama, H.; Endo, N. Long-term outcomes of an extracorporeal irradiated autograft for limb salvage operations in musculoskeletal tumours: Over ten years' observation. *Bone Jt. J.* **2019**, *101-B*, 1151–1159. [CrossRef] [PubMed]
14. Mihara, A.; Muramatsu, K.; Hashimoto, T.; Iwanaga, R.; Ihara, K.; Sakai, T. Combination of extracorporeally-irradiated autograft and vascularized bone graft for reconstruction of malignant musculoskeletal tumor. *Anticancer Res.* **2020**, *40*, 1637–1643. [CrossRef]
15. Roque, P.J.; Mankin, H.J.; Malchau, H. Proximal femoral allograft: Prognostic indicators. *J. Arthroplasty* **2010**, *25*, 1028–1033. [CrossRef]
16. Takeuchi, A.; Yamamoto, N.; Hayashi, K.; Matsubara, H.; Miwa, S.; Igarashi, K.; Tsuchiya, H. Joint-preservation surgery for pediatric osteosarcoma of the knee joint. *Cancer Metastasis Rev.* **2019**, *38*, 709–722. [CrossRef]
17. Picci, P.; Böhling, T.; Bacci, G.; Ferrari, S.; Sangiorgi, L.; Mercuri, M.; Ruggieri, P.; Manfrini, M.; Ferraro, A.; Casadei, R.; et al. Chemotherapy-induced tumor necrosis as a prognostic factor in localized Ewing's sarcoma of the extremities. *J. Clin. Oncol.* **1997**, *15*, 1553–1559. [CrossRef]
18. Weisstein, J.S.; Goldsby, R.E.; O'Donnell, R.J. Oncologic approaches to pediatric limb preservation. *J. Am. Acad. Orthop. Surg.* **2005**, *13*, 544–554. [CrossRef]
19. Lim, Z.; Strike, S.A.; Puhaindran, M.E. Sarcoma of the lower limb: Reconstructive surgeon's perspective. *Indian J. Plast. Surg.* **2019**, *52*, 55–61. [CrossRef]
20. Finn, H.A.; Simon, M.A. Limb-salvage surgery in the treatment of osteosarcoma in skeletally immature individuals. *Clin. Orthop. Relat. Res.* **1991**, 108–118. [CrossRef]
21. Herring, J.A. *Tachdjian's Pediatric Orthopaedics: From the Texas Scottish Rite Hospital for Children*, 3rd ed.; Herring, J.A., Ed.; Saunders: Philadelphia, PA, USA, 2002.
22. Muscolo, D.L.; Ayerza, M.A.; Aponte-Tinao, L.; Farfalli, G. Allograft reconstruction after sarcoma resection in children younger than 10 years old. In Proceedings of the Clinical Orthopaedics and Related Research; Springer: New York, NY, USA, 2008; Volume 466, pp. 1856–1862.
23. Soriani, A.; Strigari, L.; Petrongari, M.G.; Anelli, V.; Baldi, J.; Salducca, N.; Biagini, R.; Zoccali, C. The advantages of carbon fiber-based orthopedic devices in patients who have to undergo radiotherapy: An experimental evidence. *Acta Biomed.* **2020**, *91*, 1–12. [CrossRef]
24. Bagheri, Z.S.; El Sawi, I.; Schemitsch, E.H.; Zdero, R.; Bougherara, H. Biomechanical properties of an advanced new carbon/flax/epoxy composite material for bone plate applications. *J. Mech. Behav. Biomed. Mater.* **2013**, *20*, 398–406. [CrossRef] [PubMed]

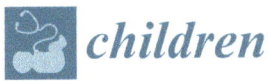

Article

Sport Ability during Walking Age in Clubfoot-Affected Children after Ponseti Method: A Case-Series Study

Vito Pavone [1,*], Andrea Vescio [1], Alessia Caldaci [1], Annalisa Culmone [1], Marco Sapienza [1], Mattia Rabito [1], Federico Canavese [2] and Gianluca Testa [1]

[1] Department of General Surgery and Medical Surgical Specialties, Section of Orthopaedics and Traumatology, University Hospital Policlinico "Rodolico-San Marco", University of Catania, 95123 Catania, Italy; andreavescio88@gmail.com (A.V.); alessia.c.92@hotmail.it (A.C.); annalisa.culmone@libero.it (A.C.); marcosapienza09@yahoo.it (M.S.); mattia.rabito@gmail.com (M.R.); gianpavel@hotmail.com (G.T.)

[2] Department of Pediatric Orthopedic Surgery, Jeanne de Flandre Hospital, Lille University Centre, 59000 Lille, France; canavese_federico@yahoo.fr

* Correspondence: vitopavone@hotmail.com

Abstract: Background: The Ponseti method (PM) of manipulative treatment for congenital talipes equinovarus (CTEV) or clubfoot became widely adopted by pediatric orthopedic surgeons at the beginning of the mid-1990s with reports of long-term successful outcomes. Sports are crucial for children's development and for learning good behavior. This study aimed to evaluate the sports activity levels in children treated with PM and to assess the different outcomes, according to gender and bilaterality. Methods: A total of 25 patients (44 feet) with CTEV treated by the PM were included in the study. The patients were clinically evaluated according to the Clubfoot Assessment Protocol, American Orthopedic Foot and Ankle Society, Ankle–Hindfoot score, the Foot and Ankle Disability Index (CAP, AOFAS, and FADI, respectively), and FADI Sport scores. Results: The overall mean CAP, AOFAS, FADI, and FADI Sport scores were 97.5 ± 6.4 (range 68.75–100), 97.5 ± 5.8 (range 73.00–100), 99.9 ± 0.6 (range 97.1–100), and 100, respectively. Gender and bilaterality did not affect outcome ($p > 0.05$). Conclusions: The data confirmed good-to-excellent outcomes in children with CTEV managed by PM. No limitations in sport performance or activity could be observed. In particular, male and female patients and patients with unilateral or bilateral involvement performed equally well.

Keywords: clubfoot; CTEV; sport; sport practice; sport activity level; young athletes; ponseti method

1. Introduction

Congenital talipes equinovarus (CTEV) is one of the most common congenital pediatric orthopedic deformities and is characterized by dorsal hyperflexion of the foot, varus of the hindfoot, forefoot adduction and increased plantar arch [1]. Clinical manifestations may depend on etiology [1], severity, and clinical course [2,3], and different treatment options are available to treat patients with CTEV [4–8].

The Ponseti method (PM) of manipulative treatment for CTEV became widely adopted by pediatric orthopedic surgeons beginning in the mid-1990s, with reports of long-term successful outcomes [9,10]. PM consists of a series of specific manipulations and cast applications to concurrently correct the forefoot, midfoot, and subtalar components of the deformity; a percutaneous Achilles tenotomy is often needed to correct the equinus component. Correction is then maintained for the first few years using a foot abduction orthosis at night and during naps. The aim of the procedure is to achieve a pain-free supple plantigrade foot with a minimal amount of surgery as practicably possible as long-term studies on the outcomes of surgical releases have reported high rates of painful and stiff feet with poor post-surgical functional outcomes [6–10].

Sport activities are crucial for children's development and for learning good behavior [11–15]. During childhood, sports may prevent future pathologies, and these activities are essential for the social inclusion and psychological well-being of the child [16–18]. Moreover, it has been shown that young sport practitioners have improved quality of life [11], brain cortical excitability [12], long-term neural adaptation mechanisms, and visuo-spatial capacities [14].

Compared to other techniques, the PM has been shown to preserve motor activities and to allow almost normal motor gross function development of children with CTEV [19,20]. In particular, Debra et al. [21] have shown a minimal delay (1.5 months) in gross motor milestone achievement, and Lohle-Akkersdijk et al. [22] reported a slight decrease in the walking speed of children with CTEV. Additionally, some authors have found that children with bilateral CTEV have worse balance and body coordination than patients with a unilateral deformity [20,23]. A few studies have assessed the sports abilities in CTEV-affected patients treated with different procedures, and PM was noted as the most effective in preserving good sports performances [10,23].

The main objective of this study was to evaluate the sports activity levels in children with CTEV managed by PM. The secondary aim was to evaluate whether any differences in sport activity performance exist between male and female patients with unilateral or bilateral CTEV; it was hypothesized that children with CTEV treated by PM have good functional outcomes and good sports activity performances regardless of gender and bilaterality.

2. Materials and Methods

2.1. Sample Eligibility Criteria

Between 2010 and 2020, 79 children with CTEV were treated with PM at the Section of Orthopaedics and Traumatology, University Hospital Policlinico "Rodolico-San Marco", University of Catania, Catania.

Inclusion criteria consisted of several requirements: (1) confirmed diagnosis of idiopathic CTEV (Forefoot adductus, midfoot cavus, hindfoot varus, hindfoot equinus); (2) initial treatment according to the PM; (3) patients > 3 years of age; (4) sports activities at a recreational or occasional level; and (5) > 2 years of follow-up.

Exclusion criteria consisted of several parameters: (1) non-idiopathic CTEV; (2) patients with underlying neurological or neuromuscular condition; (3) patients < 3 years of age; (4) no participation in sports activities; and (5) follow-up < 2 years.

According to inclusion and exclusion criteria, 36 patients were considered eligible for the study, while 11 patients were lost to follow-up and were excluded from the analysis (30.6%). A total of 44 CTEV in 25 patients were retrospectively reviewed and included in the present study.

All patients provided an informed consent to participate in the present investigation. This study was carried out according to the guidelines for Good Clinical Practice and the Declaration of Helsinki.

2.2. Ponseti Method Treatment Protocol

PM [7] consists of weekly sessions of manipulations and long-leg plaster casts with the knee at 90° of flexion. The methods onset has been described since the first weeks of life [4]. The manipulations should abduct the forefoot around the talus after the latter has been stabilized as well as mobilize the feet gently in all planes and should regularly stimulate lateral peroneal muscles in order to prevent internal rotation [4]. The first step of the cast treatment is to correct the cavus by supinating the forefoot to restore the correct arch of the foot. Subsequently, the foot is progressively abducted around the talus. Last, the equinus is corrected by dorsiflexing the foot. If the dorsiflexion of the ankle remains below 10°, percutaneous Achilles' tenotomy is performed in the operating room under general anesthesia. Following Achilles' tenotomy, a long leg cast is applied for 3 weeks, with feet externally rotated and knee flexed at 90°; after cast removal, feet are placed in splints with 60° to 70° of external rotation. The splints are worn 23 hours a day during the 3 month period, after which time they are only worn during naps and at night until age five years. Clinical follow-up is performed every six months until six years of age.

2.3. Clinical Assessment

Clinical and functional outcome were evaluated in patients with at least 2 years of follow-up by using the Clubfoot Assessment Protocol [24], the American Orthopedic Foot and Ankle Society Ankle–Hindfoot score [25], the Foot & Ankle Disability Index (CAP, AOFAS, and FADI, respectively) and FADI Sport scores [26].

The CAP contains 22 items divided into four sub-groups: (1) mobility (eight items), (2) muscle function (three items), (3) morphology (four items), and (5) motion quality I and II (seven items). The scoring is divided systematically in proportion to what is regarded as normal variation and its supposed impact on perceived physical function ranging from 0 (severe reduction/no capacity) to 4 (normal). Score grading can vary between three and five levels, and it can be used with sufficient reliability during the first seven years of childhood (it is age-independent) by examiners with good clinical experience [24].

The AOFAS Ankle-Hindfoot score consists of nine items under three different categories: (1) pain (40 points), (2) functional aspect (50 points), and (3) alignment (10 points), totaling 100 points. Items on pain and functional limitation are answered by the patient, while the alignment items are answered by an examiner [25].

The FADI is a region-specific self-reporting scale of function that includes 34 items divided into two subscales: (1) the first (FADI) consists of 26 items about activities of daily living (ADL) and pain and (2) the second (FADI Sport) consists of eight items about sports activities. Higher scores represent higher levels of function for each subscale. The ADL and sports subscales are scored separately [26].

Clinical assessment data were collected and analyzed by two authors.

2.4. Statistical Analysis

Continuous data are presented as means and standard deviations as appropriate. The Student's t-test was used to evaluate the mean and standard deviation between subgroups. Chi-square tests were used to verify the homogeneity of the group. Pearson's correlation coefficient was used to assess the correlation between the clinical scores and CTEV severity according to Pirani Score or the cast number.

The selected threshold for statistical significance was $p < 0.05$. All statistical analyses were performed using the 2016 GraphPad Software (GraphPad Inc., San Diego, CA, USA).

3. Results

3.1. Sample

The cohort of 25 patients (44 feet) consisted of 19 male (76%) and six female (24%) patients, and the mean age at time of evaluation was 6.4 ± 2.5 years (range 3–12). Eighteen patients had a bilateral (75%), and six unilateral CTEV (three left and three right).

The mean age at start of treatment was 17.2 ± 10.7 days (range 14–48). All patients had clinical follow-up for at least two years (mean: 4.6 ± 2.4 years; range 2.9–11.8). The mean number of casts per patient was 6.7 ± 1.9 (range 5–10) and 36 out of 44 feet underwent percutaneous Achilles tenotomy under general anesthesia (82%). The mean activities of daily living (ADL) Pirani's score at the beginning of treatment was 4.9 ± 1.0 (range 3–6) for included patients. If orthopedic treatment was ineffective, and feet showed no improvement, further surgery was performed. Overall, tibialis anterior transfer was performed in 1/44 feet (2.3%); no cases of posterior or medial release were recorded. Sports in which children participated included fitness (14 cases; 56.0%), soccer (four; 16%), swimming (four; 16.0%), and other activities (three; 12%), as shown in Table 1.

Table 1. Group demographics.

Group	Patients	Gender		Mean Age (Years)
		M	F	
Sample	25	19	6	6.4 ± 2.5
Unilateral	6	4	2	6.5 ± 2.3
Bilateral	19	15	4	6.4 ± 2.6

M = male; F = female.

3.2. Clinical Assessment

According to the CAP questionnaire, the mean recorded score was 97.5 ± 6.4 (range 68.75–100). Similarly, the average AOFAS was 97.5 ± 5.8 (range 73.00–100), and the average FADI score was 99.9 ± 0.6 (range 97.1–100). The average FADI Sport score for the whole cohort of patients was 100 (Table 2).

Table 2. Clinical assessment. Results reported in mean and standard deviation.

Group	Patients	CAP	AOFAS	FADI	FADI Sport
Sample	25	97.5 ± 6.4	97.5 ± 5.8	99.9 ± 0.6	100 ± 0.0
Unilateral	6	99.6 ± 0.6	100 ± 0.0	100 ± 0.0	100 ± 0.0
Bilateral	19	97.2 ± 6.9	97.1 ± 6.2	99.8 ± 0.7	100 ± 0.0
p Uni vs Bil		0.41	0.27	0.50	1.00
Male	19	97.2 ± 6.9	97.1 ± 6.5	99.8 ± 0.7	100 ± 0.0
Female	6	99.2 ± 1.6	99.2 ± 1.9	100 ± 0.0	100 ± 0.0
p Male vs Fem		0.49	0.45	0.50	1.00

Uni = Unilateral; Bil = Bilateral; CAP = Clubfoot Assessment Protocol; AOFAS = American Orthopedic Foot and Ankle Society (AOFAS) Ankle-Hindfoot score; FADI = Foot & Ankle Disability Index.

3.3. Clinical Assessment: Gender Comparison

Male and female patients had mean CAP scores of 97.2 ± 6.9 and 99.2 ± 1.6, respectively ($p = 0.49$). Similarly, no statistically significant differences could be recorded with the AOFAS score), with mean values of 97.1 ± 6.5 and 99.2 ± 1.9 for males and females, respectively ($p = 0.45$). The mean FADI score was 99.8 ± 0.7 and 100 in males and females, respectively ($p = 0.5$). The mean FADI Sport score of the whole cohort was 100 ($p = 1$), as shown in Table 2.

3.4. Clinical Assessment: Side Comparison

No statistically significant differences could be identified in the mean CAP score of unilateral clubfoot (99.6 ± 0.6) versus bilateral (97.2 ± 6.9) CTEV ($p = 0.41$). According to the AOFAS score, the mean was 100 and 97.1 ± 6.2 for unilateral and bilateral involvement, respectively ($p = 0.27$). The average FADI score was 100 ± 0.0 and 99.8 ± 0.7 in unilateral and bilateral cases, respectively ($p = 0.5$). Both groups reported a mean FADI Sport score of 100 ($p = 1$), as shown in Table 2.

3.5. Clinical Assessment and Correlations

No statistical correlation between the scores and CTEV severity according to the initial Pirani Score ($p > 0.05$) was found. Between the scores and applied cast numbers, no statistical correlation ($p > 0.05$) was recorded. The correlations data are reported in Table 3.

Table 3. Clinical assessment and correlations.

Correlation PCC (95% CI)	CAP	AOFAS	FADI	FADI Sport
Clinical scores and Pirani Score	−0.07 (−0.27; 0.14)	−0.05 (−0.26; 0.16)	−0.10 (−0.30; 0.11)	0.00 (−0.27; 0.27)
Clinical scores and Casts Number	−0.07 (−0.14; 0.27)	0.05 (−0.16; 0.26)	−0.02 (−0.38; 0.02)	0.00 (−0.27; 0.27)

PCC = Pearson Correlation Coefficient; CI = confidence interval; Uni = Unilateral; Bil = Bilateral; CAP = Clubfoot Assessment Protocol; AOFAS = American Orthopedic Foot and Ankle Society (AOFAS) Ankle-Hindfoot score; FADI = Foot & Ankle Disability Index.

4. Discussion

Patients with CTEV treated with the PM have shown excellent functional outcome at mid- and long-term evaluation periods. At the same time, good-to-excellent sports performances were found among the included patients. In particular, no differences in functional outcome or sports activity performances could be identified when comparing male and female subjects or patients with unilateral and bilateral CTEV. Several articles have reported good outcome in patients with CTEV managed by the PM [6,27–30]. However, the literature is lacking in studies investigating the sports activity levels in children with CTEV during walking age.

Recent data highlight that patients with CTEV managed by the PM had better sports performances when compared with patients managed by other techniques [10,23]. In 2017, a clinical trial compared the sports performances of children treated by Bösch method, the Cincinnati procedure, and PM. The authors found that children managed by the PM experienced less difficulty and less pain when participating in sports compared to patients treated with other methods [10]. In addition, according to three-dimensional (3D) gait analysis, patients treated by PM had better running speed/agility ($p = 0.019$), body coordination ($p = 0.038$), and strength ($p = 0.007$) compared to patients treated with the French Functional Physical Therapy method [23].

Two studies compared the athletic abilities of children with CTEV, and compared them with the general population [31,32]. Kenmoku et al. [31] assessed 30 children with CTEV treated with PM at a mean age of 9.2 ± 1.9 years (range 7–12); all patients had an excellent Ponseti functional score and any difference between individuals with CTEV and the general population could be identified for the 50 meter run, standing long jump, 20-m shuttle meter run, repetition side steps, and sit-ups. The mere inconsistency highlighted by the authors is a different podalic pattern of the center of pressure during the walk and the running. Mir et al. [32] prospectively evaluated 48 children with CTEV using the Roye Disease Specific Index and the Physical Activity Questionnaire-Elementary School (PAC-ES) adjusted to the Irish population. Almost all included patients (97%) were able to participate in school-based physical education activities. Furthermore, all patients participated in extra-curricular sporting activities; 80% participated with a frequency of 4 to 7 days per week compared to 17% of the general population. The authors concluded that sporting participation of patients with idiopathic CTEV managed by the PM was excellent, especially for extracurricular activities.

Our study examined 25 patients with a mean age of 6.4 ± 2.5 years (range 3–12) at the time of the evaluation; the whole sample presented excellent results according to specific CTEV evaluation and sport activities in addition to specific foot and ankle assessments. The cohort highlights a good correction of the foot, and only one patient required additional surgery (tibialis anterior transfer; 2.3%) although sport participation was not negatively affected. To evaluate the sports abilities and performances of the children, the FADI Sport, a specific questionnaire consisting of eight items about sports activities, was chosen. The score assesses running, landing, lateral movements, ability to perform activities with normal technique, jumping, squatting and stopping quickly, low-impact activities, and ability to participate in desired sports with no limitations. In each of these items, the maximum rating was observed.

Mir et al. [32] reported outcomes of 16 and 19 patients with bilateral and unilateral CTEV, respectively, but did not compare these two subgroups. To the best of our knowledge, our study is the first one to investigate possible athletic ability differences according to gender and bilaterality. No differences were found in the comparison between the different subgroups. Males and females had excellent functional outcomes and could perform the preferred activity without any limitations. Similarly, patients with unilateral and bilateral CTEV have similar sport performances despite the reduced size of the affected calf [33]. Moreover, no correlations were found between the clinical scores and CTEV severity according to Pirani Score or the cast number.

Debra et al. [21] showed a minimal delay (1.5 months) in gross motor milestone achievement, and Lohle-Akkersdijk et al. [22] reported a slight decrease in walking speed of children with CTEV. Additionally, some authors found that children with bilateral CTEV have worse balance and body coordination than patients with unilateral deformities [20,23]. It could be hypothesized that these findings are related to the use of braces/splints during the early years of life. During the growing age, the progressive reduction of brace/splint time per day and the progressive involvement of children in different school, social, and sports activities may contribute to improved functional and athletic performance.

Several limitations in the analysis of our results can be described. First, this study was a single-center retrospective study, the number of patients was relatively small, and no control group was used. However, we are able to offer some evidence on outcomes of sport performance of children with CTEV treated by the PM. Moreover, patients were not followed until skeletal maturity; thus, some feet issues could potentially recur, and some patients may become symptomatic with a subsequent decrease in sports performances. Therefore, it is possible that a longer multicenter follow-up study might be necessary to predict the long-term outcome of this specific treatment option.

5. Conclusions

In conclusion, the data confirmed good-to-excellent outcomes in children with CTEV managed by PM. No limitations in sports performances or activities could be observed. In particular, male and female patients, and patients with unilateral or bilateral involvement, perform equally well.

Author Contributions: Conceptualization, A.V. and G.T.; methodology, A.V.; software, A.C. (Alessia Caldaci); validation, V.P. and G.T.; formal analysis, M.S.; investigation, M.R.; resources, A.C. (Annalisa Culmone).; data curation, M.R.; writing—original draft preparation, A.V.; writing—review and editing, G.T.; visualization, F.C.; supervision, V.P.; project administration, V.P.; funding acquisition, V.P. All authors have read and agreed to the published version of the manuscript.

Funding: This research received no external funding.

Institutional Review Board Statement: The study was conducted according to the guidelines of the Declaration of Helsinki and approved by the Institutional Review Board A.O.U. Policlinico "G.Rodolico -San Marco" of Catania (protocol code 117/2020/PO, 14 October 2020).

Acknowledgments: Thanks to our casting team.

Conflicts of Interest: The authors declare no conflict of interest.

References

1. Pavone, V.; Chisari, E.; Vescio, A.; Lucenti, L.; Sessa, G.; Testa, G. The etiology of idiopathic congenital talipes equinovarus: A systematic review. *J. Orthop. Surg. Res.* **2018**, *13*, 206. [CrossRef]
2. Wainwright, A.M.; Auld, T.; Benson, M.K.; Theologis, T.M. The classification of congenital talipes equinovarus. *J. Bone Joint Surg. Br.* **2002**, *84*, 1020–1204. [CrossRef]
3. Pavone, V.; Bianca, S.; Grosso, G.; Pavone, P.; Mistretta, A.; Longo, M.R.; Marino, S.; Sessa, G. Congenital talipes equinovarus: An epidemiological study in Sicily. *Acta Orthop.* **2012**, *83*, 294–298. [CrossRef]

4. Dimeglio, A.; Canavese, F. The French functional physical therapy method for the treatment of congenital clubfoot. *J. Pediatric Orthop. B* **2012**, *21*, 28–39. [CrossRef]
5. Utrilla-Rodríguez, E.; Munuera-Martínez, P.V.; Albornoz-Cabello, M. Treatment of clubfoot with the modified Copenhagen method: A 10-year follow-up. *Prosthet. Orthot. Int.* **2018**, *42*, 328–335. [CrossRef]
6. Pavone, V.; Testa, G.; Costarella, L.; Pavone, P.; Sessa, G. Congenital idiopathic talipes equinovarus: An evaluation in infants treated by the Ponseti method. *Eur. Rev. Med. Pharmacol. Sci.* **2013**, *17*, 2675–2679. [PubMed]
7. Ponseti, I.V.; Cummings, R.J.; Davidson, R.S.; Armstrong, P.F.; Lehman, W.B. The ponseti technique for correction of congenital clubfoot. *J. Bone Jt. Surg.* **2002**, *84*, 1889–1891. [CrossRef] [PubMed]
8. Dimeglio, A.; Canavese, F. Management of resistant, relapsed, and neglected clubfoot. *Curr. Orthop. Pract.* **2013**, *24*, 34–42. [CrossRef]
9. Herzenberg, J.E.; Radler, C.; Bor, N. Ponseti versus traditional methods of casting for idiopathic clubfoot. *J. Pediatric Orthop.* **2002**, *22*, 517–521. [CrossRef] [PubMed]
10. Švehlík, M.; Floh, U.; Steinwender, G.; Sperl, M.; Novak, M.; Kraus, T. Ponseti method is superior to surgical treatment in clubfoot–Long-term, randomized, prospective trial. *Gait Posture* **2017**, *58*, 346–351. [CrossRef] [PubMed]
11. Coledam, D.H.C.; Ferraiol, P.F. Engagement in physical education classes and health among young people: Does sports practice matter? A cross-sectional study. *Sao Paulo Med. J.* **2017**, *135*, 548–555. [CrossRef] [PubMed]
12. Päivärinne, V.; Kautiainen, H.; Heinonen, A.; Kiviranta, I. Relations between subdomains of physical activity, sedentary lifestyle and quality of life in young adult men. *Scand. J. Med. Sci. Sports* **2018**, *28*, 1389–1396. [CrossRef] [PubMed]
13. Pavone, V.; Vescio, A.; Di Silvestri, C.A.; Andreacchio, A.; Sessa, G.; Testa, G. Outcomes of the calcaneo-stop procedure for the treatment of juvenile flatfoot in young athletes. *J. Child. Orthop.* **2018**, *12*, 582–589. [CrossRef]
14. Monda, V.; Valenzano, A.; Moscatelli, F.; Salerno, M.; Sessa, F.; Triggiani, A.I.; Viggiano, A.; Capranica, L.; Marsala, G.; De Luca, V.; et al. Primary motor cortex excitability in karate athletes: A transcranial magnetic stimulation study. *Front. Physiol.* **2017**, *8*, 695. [CrossRef]
15. Bianco, V.; Berchicci, M.; Perri, R.L.; Quinzi, F.; Di Russo, F. Exercise related cognitive effects on sensory-motor control in athletes and drummers compared to non-athletes and other musicians. *Neuroscience* **2017**, *360*, 39–47. [CrossRef] [PubMed]
16. Holt, N.L.; Hoar, S.; Fraser, S.N. How does coping change with development? A review of childhood and adolescence sport coping research. *Eur. J. Sport Sci.* **2005**, *5*, 25–39. [CrossRef]
17. Doré, I.; Sabiston, C.M.; Sylvestre, M.P.; Brunet, J.; O'Loughlin, J.; Abi Nader, P.; Bélanger, M. Years participating in sports during childhood predicts mental health in adolescence: A 5-year longitudinal study. *J. Adolesc. Health* **2019**, *64*, 790–796. [CrossRef]
18. Romero-Ayuso, D.; Ruiz-Salcedo, M.; Barrios-Fernández, S.; Triviño-Juárez, J.M.; Maciver, D.; Richmond, J.; Muñoz, M.A. Play in children with neurodevelopmental disorders: Psychometric properties of a parent report measure 'My Child's Play'. *Children* **2021**, *8*, 25. [CrossRef]
19. Andriesse, H.; Westbom, L.; Hägglund, G. Motor ability in children treated for idiopathic clubfoot. A controlled pilot study. *BMC Pediatrics* **2009**, *9*, 78. [CrossRef] [PubMed]
20. Lööf, E.; Andriesse, H.; André, M.; Böhm, S.; Iversen, M.D.; Broström, E.W. Gross motor skills in children with idiopathic clubfoot and the association between gross motor skills, foot involvement, gait, and foot motion. *J. Pediatric Orthop.* **2019**, *39*, 359–365. [CrossRef]
21. Sala, D.A.; Chu, A.; Lehman, W.B.; van Bosse, H.J. Achievement of gross motor milestones in children with idiopathic clubfoot treated with the Ponseti method. *J. Pediatric Orthop.* **2013**, *33*, 55–58. [CrossRef]
22. Lohle-Akkersdijk, J.J.; Rameckers, E.A.; Andriesse, H.; de Reus, I.; van Erve, R.H. Walking capacity of children with clubfeet in primary school: Something to worry about? *J. Pediatric Orthop. B* **2015**, *24*, 18–23. [CrossRef] [PubMed]
23. Zapata, K.A.; Karol, L.A.; Jeans, K.A.; Jo, C.H. Gross motor function at 10 years of age in children with clubfoot following the French physical therapy method and the Ponseti technique. *J. Pediatric Orthop.* **2018**, *38*, e519–e523. [CrossRef] [PubMed]
24. Andriesse, H.; Hägglund, G.; Jarnlo, G.B. The clubfoot assessment protocol (CAP); description and reliability of a structured multi-level instrument for follow-up. *BMC Musculoskelet Disord* **2005**, *6*, 40. [CrossRef]
25. Leigheb, M.; Vaiuso, D.; Rava, E.; Pogliacomi, F.; Samaila, E.M.; Grassi, F.A.; Sabbatini, M. Translation, cross-cultural adaptation, reliability, and validation of the Italian version of the American Orthopaedic Foot and Ankle Society—MetaTarsoPhalangeal-InterPhalangeal scale (AOFAS-MTP-IP) for the hallux. *Acta Biomed.* **2019**, *90*, 118–126. [PubMed]
26. Martin, R.L.; Burdett, R.G.; Irrgang, J.J. Development of the Foot and Ankle Disability Index (FADI). *J. Orthop. Sports Phys. Ther.* **1999**, *29*, A32–A33.
27. Bina, S.; Pacey, V.; Barnes, E.H.; Burns, J.; Gray, K. Interventions for congenital talipes equinovarus (clubfoot). *Cochrane Database Syst. Rev.* **2020**, *5*, CD008602.
28. Goksan, S.B. Treatment of congenital clubfoot with the Ponseti method. *Acta Orthop. Traumatol. Turc.* **2002**, *36*, 281–287.
29. Segev, E.; Keret, D.; Lokiec, F.; Yavor, A.; Wientroub, S.; Ezra, E.; Hayek, S. Early experience with the Ponseti method for the treatment of congenital idiopathic clubfoot. *Isr. Med. Assoc. J.* **2005**, *7*, 307–310.
30. Abdelgawad, A.A.; Lehman, W.B.; Van Bosse, H.J.; Scher, D.M.; Sala, D.A. Treatment of idiopathic clubfoot using the Ponseti method: Minimum 2-year follow-up. *J. Pediatric Orthop B* **2007**, *16*, 98–105. [CrossRef]
31. Kenmoku, T.; Kamegaya, M.; Saisu, T.; Ochiai, N.; Iwakura, N.; Iwase, D.; Takahashi, K.; Takaso, M. Athletic ability of school-age children after satisfactory treatment of congenital clubfoot. *J. Pediatric Orthop.* **2013**, *33*, 321–325. [CrossRef] [PubMed]

32. Mir, M.; Morrissey, D.; Noel, J.; Kelly, P. Sports participation amongst children treated with the Ponseti method for Idiopathic congenital talipes equinovarus. *Physiotherapy* **2015**, *101*, e1112–e1113. [CrossRef]
33. Ippolito, E.; De Maio, F.; Mancini, F.; Bellini, D.; Orefice, A. Leg muscle atrophy in idiopathic congenital clubfoot: Is it primitive or acquired? *J. Child. Orthop.* **2009**, *3*, 171–178. [CrossRef] [PubMed]

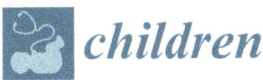

Article

Double Diapering Ineffectiveness in Avoiding Adduction and Extension in Newborns Hips

Maurizio De Pellegrin [1], Chiara Maria Damia [2], Lorenzo Marcucci [1] and Desiree Moharamzadeh [3,*]

[1] Pediatric Orthopedic Unit, San Raffaele Hospital (IRCCS Ospedale San Raffaele), 20132 Milan, Italy; depellegrin.maurizio@hsr.it (M.D.P.); lore.marcucci93@gmail.com (L.M.)
[2] Residency Program Pediatrics, Vita-Salute San Raffaele University, 20132 Milan, Italy; chiaradamia86@gmail.com
[3] Department of Orthopedic and Traumatology, San Raffaele Hospital, 20132 Milan, Italy
* Correspondence: moharamzadeh.desiree@hsr.it; Tel.: +39-02-2643-2346

Abstract: Hip flexion and abduction is fundamental for developmental dysplasia of the hip (DDH) treatment. At present, double diaper treatment has been inappropriately adopted when DDH is suspected. The aim of this study was to verify whether double diapers influence a newborn's hip position. Here, we studied 50 children (23 female; 27 male; average age 62.33 ± 20.50 days; average birth weight 3230 ± 447 g) with type I hips according to Graf. At the same time of the ultrasound (US) examination, the following hip positions were measured using a manual protractor: (1) spontaneous position, supine on the outpatient bed without a diaper; (2) spontaneous position, with a double diaper; and (3) squatting position on the caretakers' side. Statistical analysis was performed with a t-test to compare between (1) the spontaneous position without a diaper and with double diapers; (2) the spontaneous position with double diapers as well as the squatting position on the caretakers' side with a diaper. The comparison between the hip position without diaper and with double diapers was statistically not significant for all measurements, i.e., right hip flexion ($p < 0.33$), left hip flexion ($p < 0.34$), and right and left hip abduction ($p < 0.87$). The comparison between the hip position with double diapers and on the caretakers' side was statistically significant for all measurements, i.e., right hip flexion ($p < 0.001$), left hip flexion ($p < 0.001$) and right and left hip abduction ($p < 0.001$). We found that the use of double diapers did not affect hip position, while the position formed on the caretaker's side shows favorable influence.

Keywords: douple diapering; neonatal hip; DDH prevention; hip positioning; hip extension; hip adduction

Citation: De Pellegrin, M.; Damia, C.M.; Marcucci, L.; Moharamzadeh, D. Double Diapering Ineffectiveness in Avoiding Adduction and Extension in Newborns Hips. *Children* **2021**, *8*, 179. https://doi.org/10.3390/children8030179

Academic Editor: Vito Pavone

Received: 20 January 2021
Accepted: 19 February 2021
Published: 26 February 2021

Publisher's Note: MDPI stays neutral with regard to jurisdictional claims in published maps and institutional affiliations.

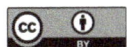

Copyright: © 2021 by the authors. Licensee MDPI, Basel, Switzerland. This article is an open access article distributed under the terms and conditions of the Creative Commons Attribution (CC BY) license (https://creativecommons.org/licenses/by/4.0/).

1. Introduction

The femoral head and the acetabulum mutually influence one another's growth and evolution starting from the prenatal period. The natural fetal position, also known as the "human position" according to Salter, refers to very flexed and moderately abducted hips. The physiological development of the hip during growth is determined by the centering of the femoral head in the acetabulum, and this is guaranteed by adequate degrees of flexion and abduction of the hips. It is known that the African populations, who culturally keep newborns in this position [1], do not observe hip dysplasia as a newborn and adult disease. On the other hand, it is well known that in countries with a cold climate, such as in Lapland, Northern China, Canada, and Japan, where for climatic reasons infants are swaddled with their lower limbs straight (and therefore with hips in extension and adduction), the risk of hip dysplasia is increased [1,2]. After a public awareness campaign was developed to eliminate these traditions, the incidence of hip dysplasia in infants dropped dramatically [2]. All treatments, past [3] and present [2,4–7], for both hip dysplasia prevention and management, point out the central concept of positioning the hips flexed and abducted to avoid opposite positions such extension and adduction.

Some health care providers identify the use of double diapers as a simple system to obtain the desired position for the correct development of the hips. In fact, although the technique is not scientifically based, double diapers are often recommended by pediatricians as a first therapeutic step during the waiting period before the instrumental procedure, which currently is the ultrasound (US) examination. It is also recommended as a treatment in cases of limited hip abduction, regardless of the US findings, or as a therapeutic alternative to other more invasive abduction splinting devices. This therapeutic indication is widespread and still suggested. Teanby reported that up to 19.3% of the population in some European countries has been treated with double diapers [8,9].

The introduction of US examination as a screening technique of developmental dysplasia of the hip (DDH) has further refined the diagnosis of dysplasia, allowing the identification of even modest alterations of the acetabulum and introducing the concept of spontaneous correction. In these hips, the double diaper treatment has been widely used as well.

In literature, double or triple diaper treatment for the management and prevention of DDH has always been mentioned, despite the demonstrated doubtful utility [10,11]. The aim of this study is therefore to evaluate whether the double diaper treatment is able to modify the spontaneous position of the newborn's hips and avoid adduction and extension.

2. Materials and Methods

Data were collected of 50 children (23 females and 27 males), who were consecutively referred to our DDH dedicated outpatient clinic for a clinical ultrasound evaluation of the hips. The clinical history of all newborns was evaluated, with regards to the fetus position during pregnancy and uterus postural anomalies, as well as the fetal anomalies diagnosed using the US examination during pregnancy, twin pregnancy, and weight at birth. The clinical examination included the evaluation of the hips regarding spontaneous posture, limitation of abduction, and the presence of clinical signs of dysplasia (Ortolani and Barlow). All newborns then underwent an US examination of the hips according to Graf [12] performed by the same operator who is certified for this method.

Inclusion criteria were as follows:

(i) single pregnancy with cephalic presentation and physiological postnatal development
(ii) no functional limitations of the hips at clinical examination, particularly those of abduction
(iii) normal range weight
(iv) infants younger than 3 months
(v) infants with type I hips at the US examination according to Graf classification (Figure 1)

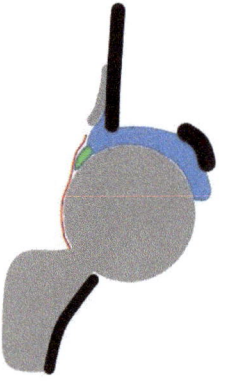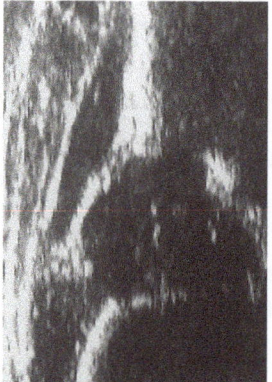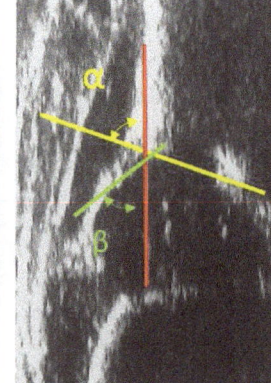

Figure 1. Normal newborn hip. Ultrasound (US) and diagram showing a type I according to Graf.

Exclusion criteria were:

(i) twins or non-cephalic presentation in pregnancy (breech, transverse) and abnormal postnatal development
(ii) infants who presented with clinical signs of dysplasia or functional limitations of the hips, particularly abduction
(iii) premature or non-normal weight newborns
(iv) infants older than 3 months
(v) infants with non-Type I hips at US examination according to Graf classification

Average age was 62.33 days (SD ± 20.50 days) and average birth weight was 3230 g (SD ± 447 g). The newborns were measured in the spontaneous position of the hips with a manual protractor [13]. The measurements were all achieved after the US examination in 3 steps: (1) supine, in spontaneous position on the outpatient bed without a diaper; (2) supine, in spontaneous position on the outpatient bed with double diapers; (3) in a squatting position on the caretakers' side, wearing a single diaper.

A statistical analysis was performed with a *t*-test in order to compare between (1) the spontaneous position without a diaper and with double diapers, and (2) the spontaneous position with double diapers as well as the squatting position on the caretakers' side with a diaper (Figures 2 and 3).

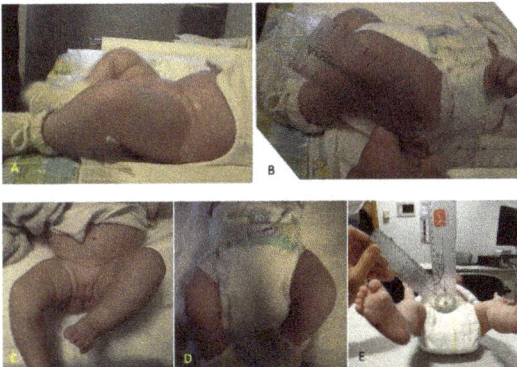

Figure 2. Hip position in a 2-month old infant: (**A**) evaluation of hip flexion without diaper; (**B**) with double diapers. Measurements with a of hip flexion angle with protractor: (**C**) evaluation of hip abduction without diaper; (**D**) with double diapers; (**E**) measurement of abduction with protractor.

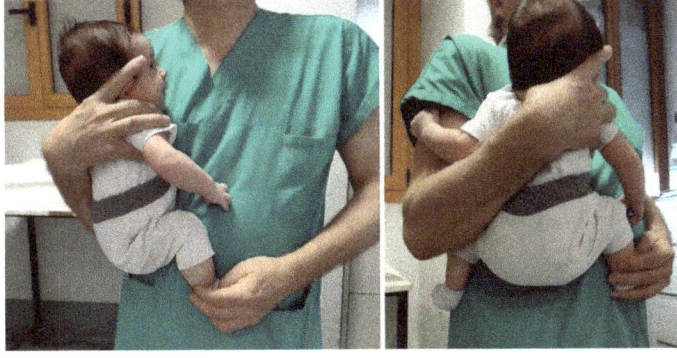

Figure 3. Hip position in a 2-month old infant when held on the caretakers' side. Flexion is approximately 100° and abduction 60°.

3. Results

Flexion and abduction measurements data of both the hips (average values and standard deviation, SD) in the spontaneous supine position of the infant on the outpatient bed without diaper, in the spontaneous position of the infant after application of double diapers, and in the squatting position on the caretakers' side with a diaper, are shown in Tables 1 and 2. The data of the statistical analysis conducted by a *t*-test for the comparison between the spontaneous position of the hips without a diaper and the spontaneous position with double diapers were statistically not significant for all measurements, i.e., right hip flexion ($p < 0.33$), left hip flexion ($p < 0.33$), right and left hip abduction ($p < 0.87$). The comparison between the spontaneous position of the hips with double diapers and the squatting position on the caretakers' side with a diaper were statistically significant ($p < 0.001$) for all measurements taken, namely for flexion and for abduction of both the right hip and the left hip (Tables 1 and 2).

Table 1. Flexion and abduction degrees measurement of the right (R) and left (L) hips with standard deviation (SD) without diaper and with double diapers.

Hips Position	Without Diaper	Double Diapers	*p* *
R Flexion Average (SD)	25.25° (18.46°)	27.5° (21.4°)	0.33
L Flexion Average (SD)	25° (18.57°)	28.64° (22.99°)	0.34
R Abduction Average (SD)	24° (8.83°)	35.06° (26.85°)	0.87
L Abduction Average (SD)	23.5° (8.75°)	34.39° (25.12°)	0.87

* *p*: Student's *t*-test

Table 2. Flexion and abduction degrees measurement of the right (R) and left (L) hip with standard deviation (SD) with double diapers and on the caretakers' side.

Hips Position	Double Diapers	Caretakers' Side	*p* *
R Flexion Average (SD)	27.5° (21.4°)	90.74° (9.97°)	< 0.001
L Flexion Average (SD)	28.64° (22.99°)	90° (10.38°)	< 0.001
R Abduction Average (SD)	35.06° (26.85°)	54.44° (10.13°)	< 0.001
L Abduction Average (SD)	34.39° (25.12°)	54.26° (9.87°)	< 0.001

* *p*: Student's *t*-test

No statistically significant difference has been reported in the hips position with double diapers and without diapers, while there is a statistically significant difference in the position of the hips of infants held on the caretakers' side compared to infants with double diapers. These do not affect the position of the hips, while the position on the caretakers' side does.

4. Discussion

At the present date, once DDH is diagnosed with an US examination, its treatment requires a specific hip position in flexion and abduction [4,5]. Flexion is known to be effective when approximately 100° is reached, given that in this position, the pressure on the acetabular region decreases and the dislocating strength of the hamstring muscles is reduced (Figure 4). The abduction favorably centers the femoral head in the acetabulum, but the concept of a "safe zone", already expressed in 1976 by Ramsey, must be observed, as it takes in consideration the danger of maximum abduction ("frog" position) on the femoral head vascular supply. Therefore, abduction must not exceed 50–60° [14]. In all the prevention strategies, the concepts expressed above regarding hip position are always considered; adduction and extension must be avoided. In 1959, Judet and Gielis specifically proposed placing the legs in abduction for DDH as a prevention measure for all newborns until 4 months of age. In the past, also in Scandinavian countries, if a clinical suspect of DDH was present, infants' hips were flexed and abducted with the Frejka splint [7]. In Italy, the studies of the pediatrician Marino Ortolani are well known. Ortolani, after identifying the worldwide clinical sign, in an epidemiologically endemic region for DDH, recommended hip flexion and abduction even where the "clunk" was absent. After this experience, the attitude of aiding the development of the hips by regular wide diapering with hips in abduction of all presumably healthy hips (essentially all children) has spread not only in Italy but also elsewhere. The abduction and flexion were obtained by means of a starched abduction towel in order to direct possible cases of dysplasia towards normal development. In particular, Klisic et al. [2,6] have precisely described the use of a suitably folded baby package, which correctly protects the hips (helping to prevent DDH) by maintaining them in mild flexion and mild abduction during the neonatal period. The study reported a significant decrease in the prevalence of congenital dislocation of the hip (from 1.3% to 0.7%) 4 years after the introduction of the Klisic method [6].

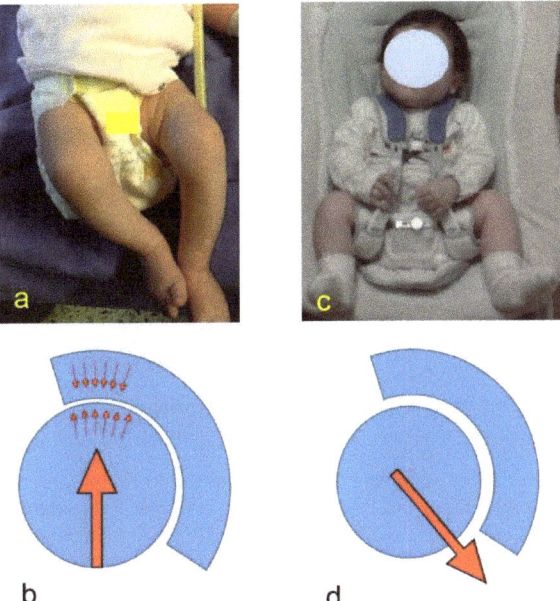

Figure 4. (**a**) Spontaneous hip position with extended and adducted hips; (**b**) diagram to note the force vector's direction (arrow) and the head's pressure on the acetabulum (small arrows); (**c**) 2-month-old infant treated with harness for developmental dysplasia of the hip (DDH), with hip flexed and abducted; (**d**) diagram to note the modified direction of the force vector.

The introduction of soft industrial diapers has considerably changed the effectiveness of the Klisic baby packages. However, the concept was maintained historically. As a matter of fact, this is the basis from which the advice of wearing double diapers as a preventive measure for DDH derives. The use of double diapers is not recommended by the American Academy of Pediatrics, which defined this therapeutic intervention as an inappropriate one and as a cause of delay in treatment (use of adequate devices) if positioned in hip dislocations [15]. The Canadian Task Force on Preventive Health Care also stated the absence of clear evidence to support the use of double or triple diapers [16]. A further study by Stephen K. Storer and David L. Skaggs confirmed no evidence of improvement of hip dysplasia when compared with non-intervention [17]. Moreover, double diapers are sometimes inappropriately seen as an alternative solution to the various abduction splints, mostly because it is considered psychologically more acceptable (Figure 4). However, no study has yet been performed where the hip position of a newborn with double diapering is objectively evaluated and in which clearly states its non-recommendation for therapeutic uses. When a DDH is diagnosed, the same problems already reported by other authors mentioned above [15–17] are also present.

The approach to this disease has dramatically changed since the introduction of US examination of the hips, used initially as a diagnostic tool and subsequently as a gold standard screening method for DDH [18]. In the past, only hip dislocations were detected and the reported incidence was 0.13%; since the introduction of US as a precise diagnostic tool that is able to show even minimal alterations of the acetabulum, the reported incidence has increased to 1.6% among the general population [19]. The US examination introduced with type IIa hips (Figure 5) the concept of physiological immaturity of the hip, which is not an expression of pathology; the hips with lower bony coverage than normal at birth (alpha angle $\geq 50°$ and $< 60°$) show in 98% of cases a spontaneous evolution towards normal bone coverage [20]. In addition, in these cases, the opinion of recommending double diapers is widespread in some European countries.

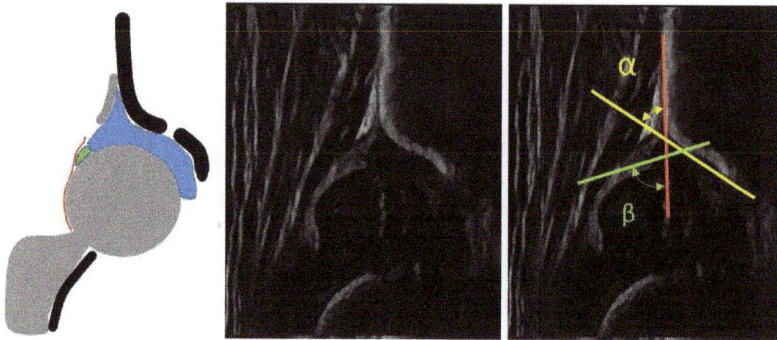

Figure 5. US image and diagram of a physiologically immature hip of a 6-week old infant. Type IIa hip according to Graf.

Thus, regarding both treatment and prevention of DDH, the real effectiveness of double diapers must still be verified, with particular attention to the real modification it can determine with respect to the position of the hip, particularly in avoiding hip adduction and extension. It is known that infants have an average hip flexion contracture of 28° at birth. The hip flexion contracture decreases to 19° at 6 weeks and to 7° at 3 months of age [21]. The measurements observed in our data without a diaper and with a double diaper do not differ significantly from these degrees of flexion. In other words, the measurement of the hips with double diapers has shown that this procedure is neither able to change the position of the hips nor guarantee the degrees of flexion and abduction necessary to achieve the correct acetabular maturation and also to avoid adduction. Our data were collected in healthy infants without functional limitations with symmetrical hip range. The ineffectiveness of double diapers is further validated in hips that already have a functional limitation, as no improvement is highlighted. Instead, the position on the caretakers' side with flexed and abducted hips is able to help in avoiding adduction and extension of the lower limbs. Obviously the requirement is that this position must be maintained constantly, which is difficult to achieve in daily life. However, the simple advice to hold infants on the side is the main idea of this study. In this regard, the current transport trends for newborns such as baby carriers and baby wrap carriers, which perhaps unknowingly respect the position of the hips described above, may be helpful and recommended for the prevention of DDH. Indeed, some recent swaddling devices must not be recommended as they imply an unfavorable hip position.

5. Conclusions

We can conclude that double diapering does not influence a newborn's hip position; the study particularly demonstrated its ineffectiveness in preventing hip adduction and extension, and it was shown to be an unfavorable position for hip development. Instead, the position on the caretakers' side or in baby carriers and baby wrap carriers, which places the hips in flexion and abduction, will favorably influence hip development.

Author Contributions: Main contributor in study design: M.D.P.; performing measurements: M.D.P.; manuscript preparation: M.D.P.; C.M.D.; L.M. and D.M. All authors have read and agreed to the published version of the manuscript.

Funding: No funding was received in the course of study, research or assembly of the manuscript.

Institutional Review Board Statement: The study was conducted according to the guidelines of the Declaration of Helsinki, and approved by the Ethics Committee of San Raffaele Hospital (Milan) (protocol PDMS-DCA, date of approval 4/03/2020).

Informed Consent Statement: Informed consent was obtained from all subjects involved in the study.

Data Availability Statement: The datasets used and/or analyzed during the current study are available from the corresponding author on reasonable request.

Conflicts of Interest: Each author certifies that he or she has no commercial associations (e.g., consultancies, stock ownership, equity interest, patent/licensing arrangements, etc.) that might pose a conflict of interest in connection with the submitted article.

References

1. Fettweis, E. Biomechanische Bedingungen der Hüftgelenksreifung. In *Das Kindliche Hüftluxations-Leiden*; Ecomed-Storck GmbH: Landsberg/Lech, Germany, 1992; pp. 52–62.
2. Price, C.T.; Ramo, B.A. Prevention of Hip Dysplasia in Children and Adults. *Orthop. Clin. North Am.* **2012**, *43*, 269–279. [CrossRef] [PubMed]
3. Judet, J.; Gielis, L. Dépistage et traitement des luxation congénitales de la hanche. *Acta Orthop. Belg.* **1959**, *25*, 440–450. [PubMed]
4. Omeroglu, H.; Kose, N.; Akceylan, A. Success of Pavlik Harness Treatment Decreases in Patients C 4 Months and in Ultrasonographically Dislocated Hips in Developmental Dysplasia of the Hip. *Clin. Orthop. Relat. Res.* **2016**, *474*, 1146–1152. [CrossRef] [PubMed]
5. Pavone, V.; Testa, G.; Riccioli, M.; Evola, F.R.; Avondo, S.; Sessa, G. Treatment of Developmental Dysplasia of Hip with Tubingen Hip Flexion Splint. *J. Pediatr. Orthop.* **2015**, *35*, 485–489. [CrossRef] [PubMed]
6. Klisic, P.; Zivanovic, V.; Brdar, R. Effects of triple prevention of CDH, stimulated by distribution of "baby packages". *J. Pediatr. Orthop.* **1988**, *8*, 9–11. [CrossRef] [PubMed]
7. Rosendahl, K.; Dezateux, C.; Aase, H.; Reigstad, H.; Alsaker, T.; Moster, D.; Markestad, T.; Fosse, K.R.; Aukland, S.M.; Lie, R.T. Immediate Treatment Versus Sonographic Surveillance for Mild Hip Dysplasia in Newborns. *Pediatrics* **2009**, *125*, e9–e16. [CrossRef] [PubMed]
8. Teanby, D.N. Ultrasound screening for congenital dislocation of the hip: A limited targeted programm. Blackburn Royal Infirmary, Lancashire, England. *J. Pediatr. Orthop.* **1997**, *17*, 202–204. [CrossRef] [PubMed]
9. Staheli, L. Management of Congenital Hip Dysplasia. *Pediatric Ann. Health Res. Prem. Collect.* **1989**, *18*, 24–32. [CrossRef] [PubMed]
10. Kotlarsky, P.; Haber, R.; Bialik, V.; Eidelman, M. Developmental dysplasia of the hip: What has changed in the last 20 years? *World J. Orthop.* **2015**, *6*, 886–901. [CrossRef] [PubMed]
11. Ergen, E.; Turkmen, E.; Ceylan, M.; Aslan, M.; Felek, S. Evaluating the effectiveness of the national hip dysplasia early diagnosis and treatment program. *Med. Sci. Int. Med. J.* **2020**, *9*, 1023. [CrossRef]
12. Graf, R. Classification of hip joint dysplasia by means of sonography. *Arch. Orthop. Trauma Surg.* **1984**, *102*, 248–255. [CrossRef] [PubMed]
13. Gripp, K.W.; Slavotinek, A.M.; Hall, J.G.; Allanson, J.E. Handbook of Physical Measurements. In *Handbook of Physical Measurements*; Oxford University Press (OUP): Oxford, UK, 2013; pp. 197–261.
14. Ramsey, P.; Lasser, S.; MacEwen, G. Congenital dislocation of the hip. Use of the Pavlik harness in the child during the first six months of life. *J. Bone Jt. Surg. Am. Vol.* **1976**, *58*, 1000–1004. [CrossRef]
15. American Academy of Pediatrics Clinical Practice Guideline: Early Detection of Developmental Dysplasia of the Hip. *Pediatrics* **2000**, *105*, 896–905. [CrossRef] [PubMed]
16. Patel, H.; The Canadian Task Force on Preventive Health Care. Preventive health care, 2001 update: Screening and management of developmental dysplasia of the hip in newborns. *CMAJ* **2001**, *164*, 1669–1677. [PubMed]
17. Storer, S.K.; Skaggs, D.L. Developmental dysplasia of the hip. *Am. Fam. Physician* **2006**, *74*, 1310–1316. [PubMed]

18. Thallinger, C.; Pospischill, R.; Ganger, R.; Radler, C.; Krall, C.; Grill, F. Long-term results of a nationwide general ultrasound screening system for developmental disorders of the hip: The Austrian hip screening program. *J. Child. Orthop.* **2014**, *8*, 3–10. [CrossRef] [PubMed]
19. O'Beirne, J.G.; Chlapoutakis, K.; Alshryda, S.; Aydingoz, U.; Baumann, T.; Casini, C.; De Pellegrin, M.; Domos, G.; Dubs, B.; Hemmadi, S.; et al. International Interdisciplinary Consensus Meeting on the Evaluation of Developmental Dysplasia of the Hip. *Ultraschall Med. Eur. J. Ultrasound* **2019**, *40*, 454–464. [CrossRef]
20. Agostiniani, R.; Atti, G.; Bonforte, S.; Casini, C.; Cirillo, M.; De Pellegrin, M.; Di Bello, D.; Esposito, F.; Galla, A.; Brunenghi, G.M.; et al. Recommendations for early diagnosis of Developmental Dysplasia of the Hip (DDH): Working group intersociety consensus document. *Ital. J. Pediatr.* **2020**, *46*, 1–7. [CrossRef] [PubMed]
21. Coon, V.; Donato, G.; Houser, C.; Bleck, E.E. Normal rages of hip motion in infant six weeks, three months, and six months of age. *Clin. Orthop. Relat. Res.* **1975**, *110*, 256–260. [CrossRef] [PubMed]

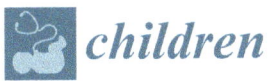

Article

Chronological Age in Different Bone Development Stages: A Retrospective Comparative Study

Abel Emanuel Moca [1], Luminița Ligia Vaida [1], Rahela Tabita Moca [2], Anamaria Violeta Țuțuianu [3,*], Călin Florin Bochiș [3,*], Sergiu Alin Bochiș [1], Diana Carina Iovanovici [4] and Bianca Maria Negruțiu [1]

[1] Department of Dentistry, Faculty of Medicine and Pharmacy, University of Oradea, 1 Universității Street, 410087 Oradea, Romania; abelmoca@yahoo.com (A.E.M.); ligia_vaida@yahoo.com (L.L.V.); bochis.alin@yahoo.com (S.A.B.); biancastanis@yahoo.com (B.M.N.)

[2] Clinical Emergency County Hospital Oradea, 37 Republicii Street, 410167 Oradea, Romania; rahelamoca@gmail.com

[3] Clinical Emergency Municipal Hospital Timișoara, 1 Hector Street, 300041 Timișoara, Romania

[4] Faculty of Medicine, University of Medicine and Pharmacy "Victor Babeș", 2 Eftimie Murgu Square, 300041 Timișoara, Romania; diana_iovanovici@yahoo.com

* Correspondence: anamaria.tutuianu7@yahoo.com (A.V.Ț.); calin_bochis@yahoo.com (C.F.B.)

Abstract: The assessment of an individual's development by investigating the skeletal maturity is of much use in various medical fields. Skeletal maturity can be estimated by evaluating the morphology of the cervical vertebrae. The aim of this study was to conduct comparisons of the chronological age in different bone development stages. The retrospective study was conducted based on lateral cephalometric radiographs belonging to patients with ages between 6 and 15.9 years, from Romania. For the assessment of skeletal maturity, the Cervical Vertebral Maturation (CVM) method was used. In total, 356 radiographs were selected, but after applying the exclusion criteria, 252 radiographs remained in the study (178 girls and 74 boys). Different mean chronological age values were obtained for the general sample, as well as for the two genders. The chronological age started to be significantly different at the CS4 stage. Patients with CS4, CS5, and CS6 stages had a significantly higher chronological age compared to patients with CS1, CS2, and CS3 stages. It was noted that patients with CS1 and CS2 stages were more frequently boys, while patients with the CS5 stage were more frequently girls.

Keywords: chronological age; skeletal maturity; Cervical Vertebral Maturation

1. Introduction

In medicine, age is essential for assessing the overall development of a patient. The chronological age, although easiest to determine if the child´s date of birth is known, often does not accurately reflect a patient´s development [1]. Various methods have been used to more precisely reproduce different developmental stages. These methods are based on determining the dental age [2] and skeletal age [3].

The assessment of skeletal maturity is useful in many fields, such as pediatrics, endocrinology [4], pediatric dentistry, and orthodontics [5]. In orthodontics, the degree of skeletal maturity influences the treatment planning and the optimal choice of treatment [6]. Hand-wrist radiographs have traditionally been used to estimate bone maturity [7], but skeletal age determination techniques based on the inspection of other bone structures have been suggested [8].

The radiological aspect of the cervical vertebrae can be used to estimate the degree of bone development. The method based on the investigation of cervical vertebrae has undergone several changes over time [9,10] and is currently known as the Cervical Vertebral Maturation (CVM) method. It involves the examination of cervical vertebrae 2, 3, and 4 on a lateral cephalometric radiograph [11]. Lateral cephalometric radiographs are necessary for establishing the diagnosis and treatment plan in orthodontics. Therefore, the assessment of skeletal maturity is possible, without any need for additional irradiation [12]. Further studies need to be conducted in order to find associations between age and CVM developmental stages.

The purpose of this study was to conduct comparisons of mean values of the chronological age in different skeletal developmental stages, for boys and girls, using the CVM method.

2. Materials and Methods

2.1. Sample Selection

This study is a retrospective and comparative radiographic study, performed on lateral cephalometric radiographs belonging to children form North-Western Romania. The lateral cephalometric radiographs were collected from three different dental private practices from the city of Oradea, Romania. The radiographs were previously used for diagnosis and treatment planning.

We included radiographs of children with ages between 6 and 15.9 years, radiographs of children for whom a signed consent form was obtained, radiographs available in a digital format, radiographs of patients with a known date of birth and known date of the radiograph, and radiographs of patients with a known gender.

Radiographs excluded from the study belonged to patients from other countries, patients with systemic diseases or genetic disorders that could impact the skeletal maturation, and patients that followed or were following an orthodontic treatment at the date when the radiographs were taken.

The selected lateral cephalometric radiographs were divided according to the gender of the patients. A total of 356 radiographs were initially selected, but after applying the exclusion criteria, only 252 were left in the study sample. The final sample consisted of 178 radiographs belonging to girls (70.6%) and 74 radiographs belonging to boys (29.4%).

2.2. Skeletal Maturity Assessment

For the assessment of skeletal maturity, the CVM method was used, as described by Baccetti et al. (2005). The CVM method consists of six different maturation stages (from CS1 to CS6), according to different morphological features of cervical vertebrae 2, 3, and 4. The inferior border of the three cervical vertebrae must be investigated, as well as the shape of the third and fourth cervical vertebrae [11].

The CVM method was applied on lateral cephalometric radiographs, available in a digital format, by examining the morphological changes of the cervical vertebrae and comparing them with the different developmental stages (Figure 1). In order to avoid inter-operator bias, the examination was performed by a single investigator (M.A.E.).

2.3. Statistical Analysis

The statistical analysis was performed by using IBM SPSS software, version 20 (IBM, Chicago, IL, USA). Quantitative variables were tested for a normal distribution by using the Shapiro–Wilk test and were expressed as the means with standard deviations, while categorical variables were expressed as counts or percentages.

The independent quantitative variables with a non-parametric distribution were tested by using a Mann–Whitney U test or Kruskal–Wallis H test. The independent quantitative variables with a parametric distribution were tested by using the One-Way ANOVA test. Categorical variables were tested by using Fisher's Exact test, and Z tests with Bonferroni correction were performed in order to further detail the results. A post-hoc Tukey HSD test and Dunn–Bonferroni test were performed in order to detail the results obtained after testing the quantitative variables.

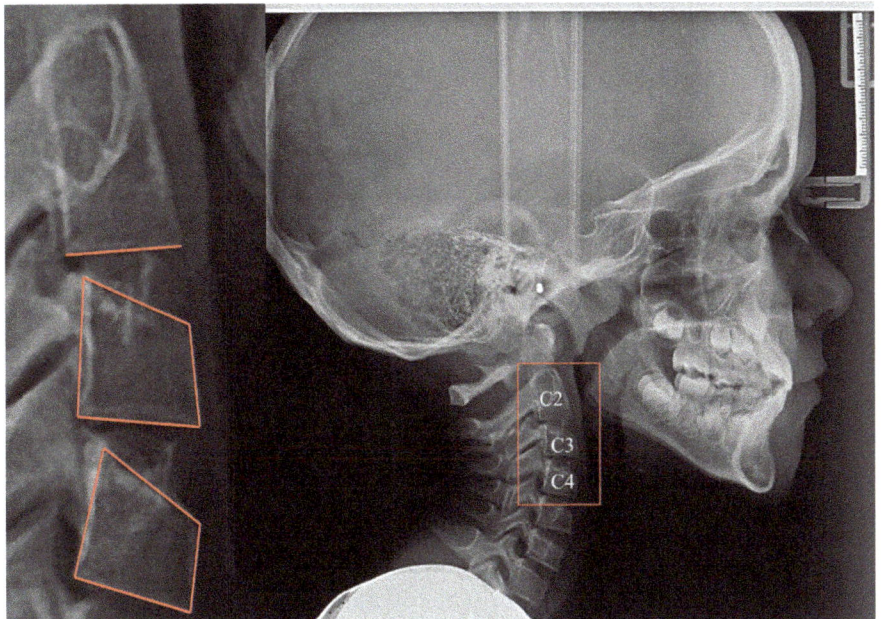

Figure 1. Lateral cephalometric radiograph with the 2, 3, and 4 cervical vertebrae highlighted.

2.4. Ethical Considerations

The study was approved by the Research Ethics Committee of the University of Oradea (No.7/15.10.2020) and was conducted in accordance with the 1964 Declaration of Helsinki and its later amendments. All radiographs belonged to patients for whom an informed consent form was previously signed by the parents.

3. Results

The mean chronological age of the patients was 11.52 ± 2.23 years, with a median (interquartile range, IQR) value of 11.65 years. The minimum age was 6.2 years and the maximum age was 15.9 years. The data in Table 1 represent the comparison of the chronological age related to the gender, with the age distribution being non-parametric in both groups, according to the Shapiro–Wilk test. The Mann–Whitney U test shows that the differences between the groups were not significant.

Table 1. Chronological age according to the gender.

Gender	Mean Age (Years) ± SD	Median (IQR)	Medium Rank	p *
Girls (p = 0.035 **)	11.535 ± 2.22	11.65 (10–13.025)	127.09	0.841
Boys (p = 0.029 **)	11.5 ± 2.29	11.65 (9.575–13.7)	125.07	

SD, standard deviation; IQR, interquartile range; * Mann–Whitney U Test; ** Shapiro–Wilk Test.

Most of the patients were distributed in the CS4 and CS5 developmental stages and the fewest were distributed in the CS2 developmental stage (Table 2). The distribution of patients according to their gender and the CVM stage revealed significant differences between the investigated groups, and –Z test with Bonferroni correction showed that the patients with CS1 and CS2 developmental stages were more frequently boys, while patients with the CS5 developmental stage were more frequently girls (Table 3).

Table 2. Distribution of the patients according to the Cervical Vertebral Maturation (CVM) stage.

CVM Stage	No.	Percentage
CS1	38	15.1%
CS2	27	10.7%
CS3	35	13.9%
CS4	64	25.4%
CS5	55	21.8%
CS6	33	13.1%

Table 3. Distribution of the patients according to their gender and CVM stage.

Gender/CVM Stage	Girls		Boys		p *
	No.	Percentage	No.	Percentage	
CS1	21	11.80%	17	23%	
CS2	14	7.90%	13	17.60%	
CS3	27	15.20%	8	10.80%	0.001
CS4	41	23%	23	31.10%	
CS5	49	27.50%	6	8.10%	
CS6	26	14.60%	7	9.50%	

* Fisher´s Exact Test.

The data in Tables 4 and 5 represent the comparison of the chronological age related to the CVM stages. The age distribution was non-parametric for patients with CS1 and CS2 stages, according to the Shapiro–Wilk test ($p < 0.05$). According to the Kruskal–Wallis H test, the differences were significant ($p < 0.001$), and the post-hoc tests showed the slow increase of the chronological age in relation to the increase of the CVM stage. The chronological age started to be significantly different at the CS4 stage. In the studied sample, the chronological age was not significantly different ($p > 0.05$) between patients with CS1, CS2, and CS3 stages. Patients with CS4, CS5, and CS6 stages had a significantly higher chronological age compared to patients with CS1, CS2, and CS3 stages, according to the post-hoc test ($p < 0.01$). Among patients with CS4, CS5, and CS6 stages, the chronological age was only significantly different between patients with CS4 and CS6 stages, and patients with CS6 stages had a significantly higher chronological age ($p = 0.002$).

Table 4. Comparison of the chronological age in different CVM stages.

CVM Stage	Mean Age (Years) ± SD	Median (IQR)	Medium Rank	p *
CS1 ($p = 0.752$ **)	9.055 ± 1.51	8.9 (7.87–10.15)	48.62	
CS2 ($p = 0.173$ **)	10.11 ± 1.59	10.1 (8.8–11.6)	77.8	
CS3 ($p = 0.700$ **)	10.35 ± 1.75	10.2 (9–11.4)	84.99	<0.001
CS4 ($p = 0.568$ **)	12.05 ± 1.73	12.05 (11–12.9)	142.62	
CS5 ($p = 0.048$ **)	12.7 ± 1.72	12.9 (11.6–13.9)	166.39	
CS6 ($p = 0.002$ **)	13.76 ± 1.35	14.1 (13.2–14.65)	202.30	

SD, standard deviation; IQR, interquartile range; * Kruskal–Wallis H Test; ** Shapiro–Wilk Test.

Table 5. Post-hoc comparison of the chronological age in different CVM stages.

CVM Stage *	CS1	CS2	CS3	CS4	CS5	CS6
CS1	-	1.000	0.498	<0.001	<0.001	<0.001
CS2	1.000	-	1.000	0.002	<0.001	<0.001
CS3	0.498	1.000	-	0.003	<0.001	<0.001
CS4	<0.001	0.002	0.003	-	1.000	0.002
CS5	<0.001	<0.001	<0.001	1.000	-	0.378
CS6	<0.001	<0.001	<0.001	0.001	0.378	-

* Dunn–Bonferroni Post-Hoc Test.

The data in Tables 6 and 7 represent the comparison of the chronological age related to the CVM stages for the girls sample, with results similar to the general sample, while the data in Tables 8 and 9 represent the comparison of the chronological age related to the CVM stages for the boys sample, which showed that the age distribution was parametric, according to the Shapiro–Wilk test ($p > 0.05$). According to the One-Way ANOVA test, the differences were significant ($p < 0.001$).

Table 6. Comparison of the chronological age in different CVM stages for girls.

CVM Stage	Mean Age (Years) ± SD	Median (IQR)	Medium Rank	p *
CS1 ($p = 0.908$ **)	8.79 ± 1.56	8.7 (7.8–10)	29.38	
CS2 ($p = 0.506$ **)	9.49 ± 1.59	9.6 (8.25–11.1)	41.36	
CS3 ($p = 0.489$ **)	10.16 ± 1.69	10.1 (9–11.3)	54.59	<0.001
CS4 ($p = 0.553$ **)	11.99 ± 1.42	12 (10.95–12.75)	98.00	
CS5 ($p = 0.076$ **)	12.57 ± 1.74	12.9 (11.5–13.7)	114.53	
CS6 ($p = 0.007$ **)	13.58 ± 1.41	14 (13.07–14.6)	139.69	

SD, standard deviation; IQR, interquartile range; * Kruskal–Wallis H Test; ** Shapiro–Wilk Test.

Table 7. Post-hoc comparison of the chronological age in different CVM stages for girls.

CVM Stage *	CS1	CS2	CS3	CS4	CS5	CS6
CS1	-	1.000	1.000	<0.001	<0.001	<0.001
CS2	1.000	-	1.000	0.006	<0.001	<0.001
CS3	1.000	1.000	-	0.010	<0.001	<0.001
CS4	<0.001	0.006	0.010	-	1.000	0.019
CS5	<0.001	<0.001	<0.001	1.000	-	0.662
CS6	<0.001	<0.001	<0.001	0.019	0.662	-

* Dunn–Bonferroni Post-Hoc Test.

Table 8. Comparison of the chronological age in different CVM stages for boys.

CVM Stage	Mean Age (Years) ± SD	Median (IQR)	p * ($p = 0.080$ ***)
CS1 ($p = 0.215$ **)	9.38 ± 1.435	9.2 (7.85–10.75)	
CS2 ($p = 0.162$ **)	10.77 ± 1.354	11.5 (9.55–11.7)	
CS3 ($p = 0.494$ **)	11.01 ± 1.9	11.5 (8.9–12.3)	<0.001
CS4 ($p = 0.398$ **)	12.15 ± 2.215	12.4 (11–14)	
CS5 ($p = 0.092$ **)	13.76 ± 1.134	14 (13.17–14.57)	
CS6 ($p = 0.792$ **)	14.42 ± 0.838	14.6 (13.7–15)	

SD, standard deviation; IQR, interquartile range; * One-Way ANOVA Test; ** Shapiro–Wilk Test; *** Levene's Test for homogeneity of variances.

Table 9. Post-hoc comparison of the chronological age in different CVM stages for boys.

CVM Stage *	CS1	CS2	CS3	CS4	CS5	CS6
CS1	-	0.246	0.241	<0.001	<0.001	<0.001
CS2	0.246	-	1.000	0.199	0.009	<0.001
CS3	0.241	1.000	-	0.582	0.044	0.003
CS4	<0.001	0.199	0.582	-	0.324	0.034
CS5	<0.001	0.009	0.044	0.324	-	0.982
CS6	<0.001	<0.001	0.003	0.034	0.982	-

* Tukey HSD Post-Hoc Test.

4. Discussion

The usefulness of the CVM method for determining the skeletal age has been suggested by many authors. Gandini et al. (2006) highlighted not only the practicality of the method, but also the low radiation dose required by lateral cephalometric radiography [13]. The CVM method seems to be able to replace the hand and wrist radiography for the estimation of bone development and can be used with confidence for this purpose [14,15]. Moreover, lateral cephalometric radiographs can be used to establish various orthodontic diagnoses [12,16], as well as to assess the morphology of other bone structures in the craniofacial region [17]. Mandibular growth can also be safely and correctly assessed on lateral cephalometric radiographs [18]. They can even be used for an evaluation of the upper airways [19]. However, when vertebral anomalies are suspected, such as osseous torticollis, examinations such as 3D-CT may be required [20].

In this study, the CVM assessment was performed manually, by direct examination of the lateral cephalometric radiographs, but computerized methods for identifying CVM stages have been developed. Vaida et al. (2019) identified the CVM stages using OnyxCeph, which is computerized software, and correlated the skeletal age of the patients with the chronological age and dental age [21]. Certain smartphone applications that allow skeletal maturity assessment based on the vertebral morphology have also been developed [22].

Most authors have found correlations between CVM stages and the chronological age. In our study, we aimed to compare the chronological age in different CVM stages and no other correlations were explored. We wanted to discover whether important differences existed between the chronological ages of various CVM stages. However, mean values of the chronological age were obtained for each CVM stage. The comparisons were conducted for the entire sample, but also, separately, for girls and boys. It was observed that the chronological age started to be significantly different starting with the CS4 stage, for the general sample, as well as for boys and girls. In other populations, correlations have been found between the skeletal age and chronological age [23]. Safavi et al. (2015) reported a positive correlation between the chronological age and all of the CVM stages in a group of Iranian girls, highlighting a moderate correlation during the circumpubertal phase. The mean chronological ages obtained for the CS4 and CS5 stages in the Iranian sample are similar to those obtained for the girls in our study. The mean chronological age in CS4 and CS5 for the Iranian sample was 11.93 and 12.66 years, respectively, while for the girls in our study, the mean chronological age in CS4 and CS5 was 12 and 12.9 years, respectively (median values) [23]. Other authors have suggested that prepubertal skeletal development may be predicted in patients with an early stage of dentition [24,25].

Some authors suggest that the chronological age is not a reliable indicator for the assessment of skeletal maturity [26].

Skeletal development can also be compared or correlated with the dental age. Różyło-Kalinowska et al. (2011) found a moderate correlation between the stages of dental development and the stages of development of the cervical vertebrae, identifying faster skeletal development for the group of female patients [27]. Faster skeletal development in female patients was also observed in our sample. The mean chronological age of the girls was generally lower than the mean chronological age of the boys for each of the CVM stages. The girls in the CS3 stage, for example, had a mean chronological age of 10.16 years, while the boys had a mean chronological age of 11.01 years. The situation is consistent for all of the CVM stages. Other authors have identified a faster development of different bone structures in female patients. Maspero et al. (2020) concluded that the development of the maxillary sinuses in girls occurred earlier than in boys, but in both genders, the development overlapped with the peak of growth [28].

Chronological age determination based on the development of the cervical vertebrae can also be used when a child´s date of birth is unknown. Mishori R. (2019) described the case of a 17-year-old boy fleeing from Honduras to the United States of America, who was initially placed in an adult facility. He was later transferred to an age-appropriate facility, after a dental exam which revealed that he was only 16–17 years old. However, age determination based on imagistic methods can be inaccurate and should be adapted in different populations [29].

5. Conclusions

The distribution of patients according to their gender and CVM stage showed significant differences between the investigated groups. Patients with CS1 and CS2 developmental stages were more frequently boys, while patients with CS5 developmental stage were more frequently girls.

In the studied sample, the chronological age was not significantly different between patients with CS1, CS2, and CS3 stages. Patients with CS4, CS5, and CS6 stages had a significantly higher chronological age compared to patients with CS1, CS2, and CS3 stages. The various mean chronological ages started to be significantly different at the CS4 stage, but differences between stages were also identified.

Author Contributions: Conceptualization, A.E.M.; methodology, A.E.M., A.V.Ț., and C.F.B.; software, R.T.M.; validation, S.A.B. and D.C.I.; formal analysis, A.V.Ț. and C.F.B.; investigation, A.E.M. and R.T.M.; resources, L.L.V. and B.M.N.; data curation, B.M.N.; writing—original draft preparation, A.E.M.; writing—review and editing, A.V.Ț., C.F.B., and B.M.N.; visualization, L.L.V.; funding acquisition, A.E.M. All authors have read and agreed to the published version of the manuscript.

Funding: This research received no external funding.

Institutional Review Board Statement: The study was conducted according to the guidelines of the Declaration of Helsinki, and approved by the Ethics Committee of the University of Oradea (No.7/15.10.2020).

Informed Consent Statement: Informed consent was obtained from all subjects involved in the study.

Data Availability Statement: The data presented in this study are available on request from the corresponding author. The data are not publicly available due to privacy reasons.

Conflicts of Interest: The authors declare no conflict of interest.

References

1. Macha, M.; Lamba, B.; Avula, J.S.S.; Muthineni, S.; Margana, P.G.J.S.; Chitoori, P. Estimation of correlation between chronological age, skeletal age and dental age in children: A cross-sectional study. *J. Clin. Diagn. Res.* **2017**, *11*, ZC01–ZC04. [CrossRef]
2. Nair, V.V.; Thomas, S.; Thomas, J.; Salim, S.F.; Thomas, D.; Thomas, T. Comparison of Cameriere's and Demirjian's methods of age estimation among children in Kerala: A pilot study. *Clin. Pract.* **2018**, *8*, 991. [CrossRef] [PubMed]
3. Christoforidis, A.; Badouraki, M.; Katzos, G.; Athanassiou-Metaxa, M. Bone age estimation and prediction of final height in patients with beta-thalassaemia major: A comparison between the two most common methods. *Pediatr. Radiol.* **2007**, *37*, 1241–1246. [CrossRef] [PubMed]
4. Martin, D.D.; Wit, J.; Hochberg, Z.; Sävendahl, L.; Van Rijn, R.R.; Fricke, O.; Cameron, N.; Caliebe, J.; Hertel, N.T.; Kiepe, D.; et al. The use of bone age in clinical practice—Part 1. *Horm. Res. Paediatr.* **2011**, *76*, 1–9. [CrossRef] [PubMed]
5. Satoh, M. Bone age: Assessment methods and clinical applications. *Clin. Pediatr. Endocrinol.* **2015**, *24*, 143–152. [CrossRef] [PubMed]
6. Durka-Zając, M.; Mituś-Kenig, M.; Derwich, M.; Marcinkowska-Mituś, A.; Łoboda, M. Radiological indicators of bone age assessment in cephalometric images. *Rev. J. Radiol.* **2016**, *81*, 347–353. [CrossRef] [PubMed]
7. Bhat, A.K.; Kumar, B.; Acharya, A. Radiographic imaging of the wrist. *Indian J. Plast. Surg.* **2011**, *44*, 186–196. [CrossRef] [PubMed]
8. Mughal, A.M.; Hassan, N.; Ahmed, A. Bone age assessment methods: A critical review. *Pak. J. Med. Sci.* **1969**, *30*, 211–215. [CrossRef] [PubMed]
9. Baccetti, T.; Franchi, L.; McNamara, J.A., Jr. An improved version of the cervical vertebral maturation (CVM) method for the assessment of mandibular growth. *Angle Orthod.* **2002**, *72*, 316–323. [CrossRef] [PubMed]
10. Franchi, L.; Baccetti, T.; McNamara, J.A., Jr. Mandibular growth as related to cervical vertebral maturation and body height. *Am. J. Orthod. Dentofac. Orthop.* **2000**, *118*, 335–340. [CrossRef] [PubMed]
11. Baccetti, T.; Franchi, L.; McNamara, J.A., Jr. The cervical vertebral maturation (CVM) method for the assessment of optimal treatment timing in dentofacial orthopedics. *Semin. Orthod.* **2005**, *11*, 119–129. [CrossRef]
12. Heil, A.; Gonzalez, E.L.; Hilgenfeld, T.; Kickingereder, P.; Bendszus, M.; Heiland, S.; Ozga, A.-K.; Sommer, A.; Lux, C.J.; Zingler, S. Lateral cephalometric analysis for treatment planning in orthodontics based on MRI compared with radiographs: A feasibility study in children and adolescents. *PLoS ONE* **2017**, *12*, e0174524. [CrossRef] [PubMed]
13. Gandini, P.; Mancini, M.; Andreani, F. A comparison of hand-wrist bone and cervical vertebral analysis in measuring skeletal maturation. *Angle Orthod.* **2006**, *76*, 984–989. [CrossRef]
14. Flores-Mir, C.; Burgess, C.A.; Champney, M.; Jensen, R.J.; Pitcher, M.R.; Major, P.W. Correlation of skeletal maturation stages determined by cervical vertebrae and hand-wrist evaluations. *Angle Orthod.* **2006**, *76*, 1–5. [CrossRef]
15. Szemraj, A.; Wojtaszek-Słomińska, A.; Racka-Pilszak, B. Is the cervical vertebral maturation (CVM) method effective enough to replace the hand-wrist maturation (HWM) method in determining skeletal maturation?—A systematic review. *Eur. J. Radiol.* **2018**, *102*, 125–128. [CrossRef]
16. Vaida, L.L.; Bud, E.S.; Halitchi, L.G.; Cavalu, S.; Todor, B.I.; Negrutiu, B.M.; Moca, A.E.; Bodog, F.D. The behavior of two types of upper removable retainers—Our Clinical Experience. *Children* **2020**, *7*, 295. [CrossRef]

17. Tepedino, M.; Laurenziello, M.; Guida, L.; Montaruli, G.; Grassia, V.; Chimenti, C.; Campanelli, M.; Ciavarella, M. Sella turcica and craniofacial morphology in patients with palatally displaced canines: A retrospective study. *Folia Morphol.* **2015**, *79*, 51–57. [CrossRef]
18. Maspero, C.; Farronato, M.; Bellincioni, F.; Cavagnetto, D.; Abate, A. Assessing mandibular body changes in growing subjects: A comparison of CBCT and reconstructed lateral cephalogram measurements. *Sci. Rep.* **2020**, *10*, 11722. [CrossRef]
19. Dobrowolska-Zarzycka, M.; Dunin-Wilczyńska, I.; Mitura, I.; Dąbała, M. Evaluation of upper airways depth among patients with skeletal class I and III. *Folia Morphol.* **2013**, *72*, 155–160. [CrossRef] [PubMed]
20. Ryoo, D.H.; Jang, D.H.; Kim, D.Y.; Kim, J.; Lee, D.W.; Kang, J.H. Congenital ossesous torticollis that mimics congenital muscular torticollis: A retrospective observational study. *Children* **2020**, *7*, 227. [CrossRef]
21. Vaida, L.L.; Moca, A.E.; Todor, L.; Țenț, A.; Todor, B.I.; Negruțiu, B.M.; Moraru, A.I. Correlations between morphology of cervical vertebrae and dental eruption. *Rom. J. Morphol. Embryol* **2019**, *60*, 175–180. [PubMed]
22. Mamillapalli, P.K.; Sesham, V.M.; Neela, P.K.; Kondapaka, V.; Mandaloju, S.P. A smartphone app for identifying cervical vertebral maturation stages. *J. Clin. Orthod.* **2015**, *49*, 582–585. [PubMed]
23. Safavi, S.M.; Beikaii, H.; Hassanizadeh, R.; Younessian, F.; Baghban, A.A. Correlation between cervical vertebral maturation and chronological age in a group of Iranian females. *Dent. Res. J.* **2015**, *12*, 443–448. [CrossRef]
24. Fernandes-Retto, P.; Matos, D.; Ferreira, M.; Bugaighis, I.; Delgado, A. Cervical vertebral maturation and its relationship to circum-pubertal phases of the dentition in a cohort of Portuguese individuals. *J. Clin. Exp. Dent.* **2019**, *11*, e642–e649. [CrossRef]
25. Franchi, L.; Baccetti, T.; De Toffol, L.; Polimeni, A.; Cozza, P. Phases of the dentition for the assessment of skeletal maturity: A diagnostic performance study. *Am. J. Orthod. Dentofac. Orthop.* **2008**, *133*, 395–400. [CrossRef]
26. Alkhal, H.A.; Wong, R.W.K.; Rabie, A.B.M. Correlation between chronological age, cervical vertebral maturation and fishman's skeletal maturity indicators in southern Chinese. *Angle Orthod.* **2008**, *78*, 591–596. [CrossRef]
27. Różyło-Kalinowska, I.; Kolasa-Rączka, A.; Kalinowski, P. Relationship between dental age according to Demirjian and cervical vertebral maturity in Polish children. *Eur. J. Orthod.* **2011**, *33*, 75–83. [CrossRef] [PubMed]
28. Maspero, C.; Farronato, M.; Bellincioni, F.; Annibale, A.; Machetti, J.; Abate, A.; Cavagnetto, D. Three-dimensional evaluation of maxillary sinus changes in growing subjects: A retrospective cross-sectional study. *Materials* **2020**, *13*, 1007. [CrossRef]
29. Mishori, R. The use of age assessment in the context of child migration: Imprecise, inaccurate, inconclusive and endangers children's rights. *Children* **2019**, *6*, 85. [CrossRef] [PubMed]

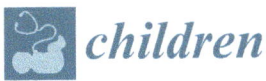

Article

Does the Duration of Each Waldenström Stage Affect the Final Outcome of Legg–Calvé–Perthes Disease Onset before 6 Years of Age?

Ho-Seok Oh, Myung-Jin Sung, Young-Min Lee, Sungmin Kim and Sung-Taek Jung *

Department of Orthopedic Surgery, National University Hospital, Gwangju 61469, Korea; koreankid07@naver.com (H.-S.O.); smj2383@naver.com (M.-J.S.); lovepoplove@naver.com (Y.-M.L.); kimsum83@gmail.com (S.K.)
* Correspondence: stjung@jnu.ac.kr

Abstract: The purpose of this study was to evaluate the outcomes of patients with Legg–Calvé–Perthes disease (LCPD) with disease onset before 6 years of age who were treated with conservative methods and to identify prognostic factors. Moreover, we evaluated the duration of the Waldenström stage and its correlation with the disease outcome. Disease severity was assessed using the lateral pillar classification, and the final outcome was evaluated using the Stulberg classification. We divided patients with LCPD into two groups according to the age at onset: group 1 (<4 years) and group 2 (4–6 years). The final outcomes of the two groups were compared. We also assessed the duration of each Waldenström stage. LCPD was noted in 49 hips of 49 patients. The lateral pillar class was A in one patient, B in 29 patients, and B/C or C in 19 patients. The Stulberg class was I or II (good) in 30 patients, III (fair) in 13 patients, and IV or V (poor) in six patients. The lateral pillar class significantly correlated with the final outcome. Groups 1 and 2 comprised 25 and 24 patients, respectively. The prevalence of good outcomes did not significantly differ between the groups ($p = 0.162$). The duration of the initial stage was 4.1 months in the good outcome group and 6.2 months in the fair or poor outcome group. The duration of the fragmentation stage of the femoral head was 5.9 months in the good outcome group and 11.9 months in the fair or poor outcome group. The durations of initial and fragmentation stages significantly differed between good outcome group and fair or poor outcome group ($p = 0.009$ and $p < 0.001$, respectively). The prognosis of patients with disease onset before the age of 6 years was favorable. The disease severity and duration of each Waldenström stage can be predictors of the outcome. Patients with prolonged initial and fragmentation stages showed worse outcomes and often required more active treatment to shorten the durations of the initial and fragmentation stages.

Keywords: Legg–Calvé–Perthes disease; Herring lateral pillar classification; Stulberg classification; Waldenström stage; duration

Citation: Oh, H.-S.; Sung, M.-J.; Lee, Y.-M.; Kim, S.; Jung, S.-T. Does the Duration of Each Waldenström Stage Affect the Final Outcome of Legg–Calvé–Perthes Disease Onset before 6 Years of Age?. *Children* 2021, 8, 118. https://doi.org/10.3390/children8020118

Academic Editor: Vito Pavone
Received: 6 January 2021
Accepted: 3 February 2021
Published: 6 February 2021

Publisher's Note: MDPI stays neutral with regard to jurisdictional claims in published maps and institutional affiliations.

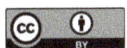

Copyright: © 2021 by the authors. Licensee MDPI, Basel, Switzerland. This article is an open access article distributed under the terms and conditions of the Creative Commons Attribution (CC BY) license (https://creativecommons.org/licenses/by/4.0/).

1. Introduction

The prognosis of Legg–Calvé–Perthes disease (LCPD) varies with the patient's age at disease onset. LCPD occurring in children under 6 years of age is usually a benign, self-limiting condition with a good outcome [1–3]. However, extensive femoral head involvement in patients with early onset is associated with a potentially poor outcome. In children under 6 years of age, the Catterall and lateral pillar classes of LCPD correlate with the prognosis [4–7].

The Waldenström classification of LCPD is based on radiographic changes over time as the disease progresses naturally. According to the classification, LCPD has four radiographic stages: initial, fragmentation, reossification, and residual [8]. In a retrospective study, the time from the first radiographic evidence of disease to the start of fragmentation was a mean of 6 (range: 1–14) months, with fragmentation and reossification stages lasting

8 (range: 2–35) and 51 (2–122) months, respectively. The disease severity positively correlated with the duration of each stage, particularly the healing stage [9]. However, few studies have attempted to correlate the duration of each stage with the outcome in younger patients [9–12].

The purpose of this study was to clarify the outcome of patients with LCPD with disease onset before 6 years of age who were treated with conservative methods, and to identify the prognostic factors, such as the age of disease onset and disease severity. Moreover, we evaluated the duration of each Waldenström stage and correlated it with the outcome.

2. Materials and Methods

Of a total of 230 hips of patients with LCPD diagnosed before 6 years of age, treated at the Chonnam National University Hospital from 1980 to 2015, 66 with adequate radiographs at presentation showed the initial stage and were followed-up until skeletal maturity. We excluded patients who were treated surgically ($n = 14$) or considered to have completely bypassed fragmentation stage ($n = 3$). Finally, we included 49 hips of 49 patients.

There were 47 boys and two girls. The patients' mean age at diagnosis was 3.9 (range: 1.9–5.9) years, and the mean follow-up duration was 14.3 (range: 6.2–27.8) years (Table 1). The medical records of all patients were reviewed to extract data on the sex, age of onset, treatment method, and follow-up duration. Moreover, two orthopedic surgeons (HSO and SK) reviewed the standard anteroposterior and frog-leg radiographs of the hips throughout the treatment course (Figure 1). To evaluate disease severity, we applied the lateral pillar classification when the disease showed maximal epiphyseal fragmentation in the fragmentation stage [12,13].

Table 1. Patient demographics.

Sex	Boy:Girl (Hips)	47:2
Location	Right:Left (hips)	24:25
Age	Average (Minimum~Maximum)	3.9 (1.9~5.9)
Follow-up duration	Average (Minimum~Maximum)	14.3 (6.2~27.8)

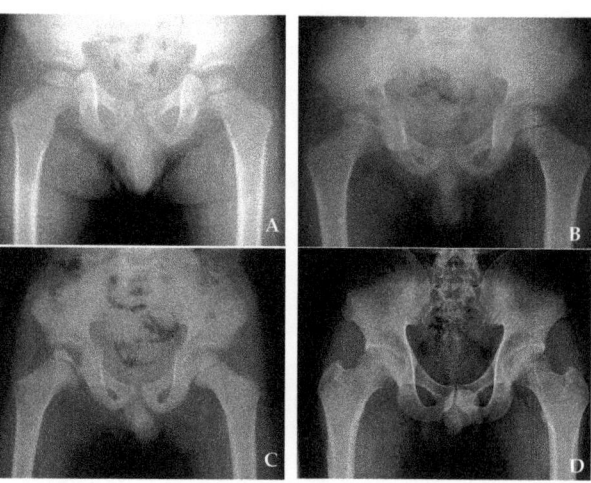

Figure 1. Anteroposterior radiograph of patients at the age of 2 years. Initial (**A**), fragmentation (**B**), reossification (**C**), and residual (**D**) stages.

To determine the Waldenström class, the interval between the first radiograph showing features of one stage and the first radiograph showing features of the next stage was determined as the duration of the stage. We used the modified Waldenström classification published by Joseph et al. [14] to determine the onset of initial, fragmentation, and reossification stages. The onset of the initial stage was defined as the time when part or whole of the epiphysis was sclerotic (Figure 1A). When one or two vertical fissures were present in the anteroposterior or frog-leg lateral view, we marked the onset of the fragmentation stage (Figure 1B). The onset of the reossification stage was defined as the time when early new bone was visible lateral to the fragmented epiphysis (Figure 1C).

The final outcome was evaluated radiographically using the Stulberg classification. The Stulberg class was determined from radiographs at the time of skeletal maturity, and patients without skeletal maturity at the final follow-up were excluded (Figure 1D) [13]. Stulberg classes I and II were considered to be good, III to be fair, and IV and V to be poor.

To evaluate whether or not age is a factor determining the prognosis of patients with LCPD before 6 years of age, we divided the patients into two groups according to the age at disease onset: group 1, <4 years of age, comprising 25 hips; and group 2, 4–6 years of age, comprising 24 hips. Both groups were compared using the Stulberg classification.

Outcomes were analyzed in terms of disease severity and age difference, with Fisher's exact probability test, using IBM SPSS statistics 21.0. Differences in the duration of each stage between the good and fair or poor outcome groups were analyzed with independent t-tests. A p-value < 0.05 was considered to be statistically significant. The kappa statistic was computed to test the inter-rater reliability of the Waldenström, lateral pillar, and Stulberg classifications. Cohen's kappa values of 0.61–0.80 were interpreted as substantial agreement, whereas values of 0.81–1.00 were interpreted as almost perfect agreement [14].

3. Results

Patients diagnosed with LCPD under the age of 6 years were classified using Herring's lateral pillar classification at the time of maximum fragmentation. Only one hip was classified as lateral pillar A and showed a good outcome (Stulberg I or II). Of 29 hips classified as lateral pillar B, 26 showed a good outcome, whereas three showed a fair outcome (Stulberg III). Of 19 hips classified as lateral pillar C, three, 10, and six showed good, fair, and poor outcomes, respectively (Stulberg IV or V; Table 2). The lateral pillar class significantly correlated with the final outcome ($p < 0.001$). Regarding agreement using Cohen's kappa, almost perfect agreement was obtained for the Herring's lateral pillar and Stulberg classifications (Cohen's kappa of 0.85 and 0.83, respectively).

Table 2. Outcome according to the lateral pillar class.

Lateral Pillar Class	Good (Stulberg Class I or II)	Fair (Stulberg Class III)	Poor (Stulberg Class IV or V)
A	1	0	0
B	26	3	0
B/C, C	3	10	6

p-value < 0.001.

Of 25 hips in group 1, 14 showed a good outcome, whereas 11 showed a fair or poor outcome. Of 24 hips in group 2, 18 showed a good outcome, whereas six showed a fair or poor outcome. There were no significant differences between the age groups in terms of the final outcome ($p = 0.162$; Table 3).

The duration of the initial stage was 4.1 months (0.7~9.8) in the good outcome group and 6.2 months (2.6~13.5) in the fair or poor outcome group. The duration of the fragmentation stage was 5.9 months (1.0~16.0) in the good outcome group and 11.9 months (4.2~23.6) in the fair or poor outcome group. The durations of both initial and fragmentation stages significantly differed between the two groups ($p = 0.009$ and $p < 0.001$, respectively; Table 4).

Regarding agreement using Cohen's kappa, substantial agreement was obtained for the Waldenström classification (Cohen's kappa of 0.77).

Table 3. Outcome according to age.

	Stulberg Class I or II	Stulberg Class III, IV, or V	p-Value
Group I (age < 4 years)	14	11	0.162
Group II (age ≥ 4 years)	18	6	

Group I (n = 25), group II (n = 24).

Table 4. Durations of the initial and fragmentation stages in each outcome group.

	Stulberg Class I or II	Stulberg Class III, IV, or V	p-Value
Initial	4.1 (0.7~9.8)	6.2 (2.6~13.5)	0.009
Fragmentation	5.9 (1.0~16.0)	11.9 (4.2~23.6)	<0.001

Mean durations of the initial and fragmentation stages were 5.0 and 8.2 months, respectively. p-value of the comparison between the durations of the initial and fragmentation stages <0.001.

4. Discussion

In recent studies, LCPD diagnosed in children less than 6 years of age has shown good final outcomes. In studies by Rosenfeld et al. [6], Gent et al. [5], and Nakamura et al. [7], 80% (131/164), 65% (45/69), and 63% (72/114) of hips showed a good final outcome (Table 5), respectively. Moreover, all these studies revealed a significant correlation between the lateral pillar class and the final outcome. Although we only included patients with skeletal maturity at the final follow-up, excluding those with complete bypass surgery, the results of our study (61.2%, 30/49 hips) were consistent with those of other studies and showed a significant correlation between the lateral pillar class and the final outcome (Table 2). These data support the idea that the overall outcome of patients diagnosed with LCPD under 6 years of age is favorable.

Table 5. Comparison of the disease severity with the final outcome in previously reported studies.

	Lateral Pillar		Stulberg		
	A or B	B/C or C	I or II	III	IV or V
Rosenfeld et al. [6]	115 (61.2)	73 (38.8)	152 (80.9)	17 (9.0)	19 (10.1)
Gent et al. [5]	39 (56.5)	30 (43.5)	45 (65)	14 (20)	10 (15)
Nakamura et al. [7]	39 (34.2)	75 (65.8)	72 (63.1)	28 (25.6)	14 (12.3)
This study	30 (61)	19 (29)	30 (61)	13 (27)	6 (12)

Many studies have suggested that the final outcome of LCPD is significantly affected by patient age at the time of disease onset. The younger the patient at onset, the milder the disease severity [1,15–17]. Presumably, this is related to one or more of the following factors: a smaller volume of infracted bone, a more abundant circulation to the proximal femoral epiphysis, and an increased ability of bone to remodel in very young children [18]. A few studies have evaluated the correlation between age and the prognosis of patients diagnosed with LCPD under 6 years of age. Rosenfeld et al. reported [6] that the combination of young age (0 to 3 years 11 months) with lateral pillar class A or B significantly correlated with a better outcome in patients diagnosed with LCPD under 6 years of age. However, Nakamura et al. reported [7] that a good outcome did not significantly differ between younger (0 to 3 years 11 months) and older groups (4 years to 5 years 11 months). In our study, in patients diagnosed with LCPD under 6 years of age treated with conservative methods, the final outcome did not significantly differ between groups 1 and 2 (Table 4).

Waldenström classified LCPD based on radiographic changes into the initial, fragmentation, reossification, and residual stages [8], and the duration of each stage varied across patients. Benjamin Joseph et al. [10] reviewed 610 patients with LCPD and divided the disease progression into seven stages (Ia, Ib, IIa, IIb, IIa, IIIb, and IV) using the modified Elizabethtown classification, which subdivides Waldenström stages. The median durations of the initial (Ia and Ib), fragmentation (IIa and IIb), and reossification (IIIa and IIIb) stages were approximately 7, 8, and 18 months, respectively. However, the duration of any disease stage did not differ significantly among the Catterall groups in their study. Herring et al. [9] also reported that the duration of the fragmentation stage of the disease was approximately 9 months. Catterall et al. [11] suggested that the disease duration varies with the final outcome, with the disease duration being 8 months shorter in children with good results compared to those with poor results. In our study, despite only including patients with LCPD onset at less than 6 years of age, the median durations of the initial and fragmentation stages were approximately 5 and 8 months, respectively, showing a shorter duration of the initial stage and similar duration of the fragmentation stage compared to other studies. The duration of the initial stage positively correlates with that of the fragmentation stage. Moreover, prolonged initial and fragmentation stages are associated with a worse prognosis. Several events occur during the fragmentation period, including subluxation of the femoral epiphysis and collapse of the lateral pillar, that increase the risk for permanent femoral head deformity [10,13]. Accordingly, the duration of the initial stage positively correlates with that of the fragmentation stage, and in such cases, even if patients with LCPD are under 6 years of age, they may require active treatment such as surgical treatment.

This study has several limitations. First, we used several subjective staging systems. Although two orthopedic surgeons reviewed the radiographs to reduce bias, the subjectivity of the staging systems could have caused a bias. Second, features that characterized each stage may have preceded the date of each radiograph, resulting in overestimation of the stage duration. Third, the number of patients included in this study was too small for an optimal statistical analysis.

5. Conclusions

In conclusion, the prognosis of patients with LCPD onset before the age of 6 years treated with conservative methods is favorable. The durations of initial and fragmentation stages can predict the outcome; in particular, prolongation of the fragmentation stage can adversely affect the prognosis. Patients with a prolonged initial stage may require active treatment to shorten the durations of the initial and fragmentation stages.

Author Contributions: Conceptualization: S.-T.J. and H.-S.O.; methodology: Y.-M.L. and S.K.; validation: S.-T.J. and S.K.; formal analysis: H.-S.O. and Y.-M.L.; investigation: H.-S.O. and M.-J.S.; data curation: M.-J.S.; writing—original draft preparation: H.-S.O. and Y.-M.L.; writing—review and editing: H.-S.O. and S.K.; visualization: M.-J.S.; supervision: S.-T.J. All authors have read and agreed to the published version of the manuscript.

Funding: No external funding was received for this study.

Institutional Review Board Statement: We conducted this study in compliance with the principles of the Declaration of Helsinki. The protocol of this study was reviewed and approved by the Institutional Review Board of the Chonnam National University Hospital (IRB No. CNUH-2016-161). Written informed consent was obtained.

Informed Consent Statement: Patient consent was waived due to retrospective nature of this study.

Data Availability Statement: The data was not publicly available due to ethical reasons and patient privacy.

Conflicts of Interest: The authors declare no conflict of interest.

References

1. Catterall, A. The natural history of perthes' disease. *J. Bone Jt. Surg. Br. Vol.* **1971**, *53*, 37–53. [CrossRef]
2. Ippolito, E.; Tudisco, C.; Farsetti, P. The long-term prognosis of unilateral Perthes' disease. *J. Bone Jt. Surg. Br. Vol.* **1987**, 243–250. [CrossRef] [PubMed]
3. Salter, R.B.; Thompson, G.H. Legg-Calve-Perthes disease. The prognostic significance of the subchondral fracture and a two-group classification of the femoral head involvement. *J. Bone Jt. Surg. Am. Vol.* **1984**, *66*, 479–489. [CrossRef]
4. Canavese, F.; Dimeglio, A. Perthes' disease: Prognosis in children under six years of age. *J. Bone Jt. Surg. Br. Vol.* **2008**, *90*, 940–945. [CrossRef] [PubMed]
5. Gent, E.; Antapur, P.; Mehta, R.L.; Sudheer, V.M.; Clarke, N.M. Predicting the outcome of Legg-Calve-Perthes' disease in children under 6 years old. *J. Child. Orthop.* **2007**, *1*, 159. [CrossRef] [PubMed]
6. Rosenfeld, S.B.; Herring, J.A.; Chao, J.C. Legg-Calvé-Perthes Disease: A Review of Cases with Onset before Six Years of Age. *J. Bone Jt. Surg. Am. Vol.* **2007**, *89*, 2712–2722. [CrossRef] [PubMed]
7. Nakamura, J.; Kamegaya, M.; Saisu, T.; Kakizaki, J.; Hagiwara, S.; Ohtori, S.; Orita, S.; Takahashi, K. Outcome of Patients With Legg-Calvé-Perthes Onset Before 6 Years of Age. *J. Pediatr. Orthop.* **2015**, *35*, 144–150. [CrossRef] [PubMed]
8. Herring, J.A. *Tachdjian's Pediatric Orthopaedics*, 3rd ed.; Saunders: Philadelphia, PA, USA, 2002; p. 675.
9. Herring, J.A.; Williams, J.J.; Neustadt, J.N.; Early, J.S. Evolution of Femoral Head Deformity during the Healing Phase of Legg-Calvé-Perthes Disease. *J. Pediatr. Orthop.* **1993**, *13*, 41–45. [CrossRef] [PubMed]
10. Joseph, B.; Varghese, G.; Mulpuri, K.; Narasimha Rao, K.; Nair, N.S. Natural evolution of Perthes disease: A study of 610 children under 12 years of age at disease onset. *J. Pediatric Orthop.* **2003**, *23*, 590–600. [CrossRef]
11. Catteral, A. Legg-Calve-Perthes' Disease. In *Current Problems in Orthopaedics*; Curchill Livingstone: Edinburgh, UK, 1982.
12. Catterall, A. Natural history, classification, and x-ray signs in Legg-Calve-Perthes' disase. *Acta Orthopaedica Belgica.* **1980**, *46*, 346–351.
13. Herring, J.A.; Kim, H.T.; Browne, R. Legg-Calve-Perthes disease. Part I: Classification of radiographs with use of the modified lateral pillar and Stulberg classifications. *J. Bone Jt. Surg. Am. Vol.* **2004**, *86*, 2103–2120. [CrossRef]
14. Cohen, J. Weighted kappa: Nominal scale agreement provision for scaled disagreement or partial credit. *Psychol. Bull.* **1968**, *70*, 213–220. [CrossRef] [PubMed]
15. Ippolito, E.; Tudisco, C.; Farsetti, P. Long-Term Prognosis of Legg-Calvé-Perthes Disease Developing During Adolescence. *J. Pediatr. Orthop.* **1985**, *5*, 652–656. [CrossRef]
16. Snyder, C.R. Legg-Perthes disease in the young hip–does it necessarily do well? *J. Bone Jt. Surg. Am. Vol.* **1975**, *57*, 751–759. [CrossRef]
17. Ingman, A.M.; Paterson, D.C.; Sutherland, A.D. A Comparison between Innominate Osteotomy and Hip Spica in the Treatment of Legg-Perthes? *Disease Clin. Orthop. Relat. Res.* **1982**, 141–147. [CrossRef]
18. Clarke, T.E.; Finnegan, T.L.; Fisher, R.L.; Bunch, W.H.; Gossling, H.R. Legg-Perthes disease in children less than four years old. *J. Bone Jt. Surg. Am. Vol.* **1978**, *60*, 166–168. [CrossRef]

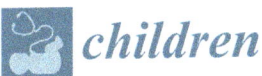

Review

Dynamic and Static Splinting for Treatment of Developmental Dysplasia of the Hip: A Systematic Review

Vito Pavone [1,*], Claudia de Cristo [1], Andrea Vescio [1], Ludovico Lucenti [1], Marco Sapienza [1], Giuseppe Sessa [1], Piero Pavone [2] and Gianluca Testa [1]

1. Department of General Surgery and Medical Surgical Specialties, Section of Orthopaedics and Traumatology, University Hospital Policlinico-Vittorio Emanuele, University of Catania, 95123 Catania, Italy; decristo.claudia@gmail.com (C.d.C.); andreavescio88@gmail.com (A.V.); ludovico.lucenti@gmail.com (L.L.); marcosapienza09@yahoo.it (M.S.); giusessa@unict.it (G.S.); gianpavel@hotmail.com (G.T.)
2. Department of Clinical and Experimental Medicine, Section of Pediatrics and Child Neuropsychiatry, University of Catania, 95123 Catania, Italy; ppavone@unict.it
* Correspondence: vitopavone@hotmail.com

Abstract: Background: Developmental dysplasia of the hip (DDH) is one of the most common pediatric conditions. The current gold-standard treatment for children under six months of age with a reducible hip is bracing, but the orthopedic literature features several splint options, and each one has many advantages and disadvantages. The aim of this review is to analyze the available literature to document the up-to-date evidence on DDH conservative treatment. Methods: A systematic review of PubMed and Science Direct databases was performed by two independent authors (C.d.C. and A.V.) using the keywords "developmental dysplasia hip", "brace", "harness", "splint", "abduction brace" to evaluate studies of any level of evidence that reported clinical or preclinical results and dealt with conservative DDH treatment. The result of every stage was reviewed and approved by the senior investigators (V.P. and G.T.). Results: A total of 1411 articles were found. After the exclusion of duplicates, 367 articles were selected. At the end of the first screening, following the previously described selection criteria, we selected 29 articles eligible for full text reading. The included articles mainly focus on the Pavlik harness, Frejka, and Tubingen among the dynamic splint applications as well as the rhino-style brace, Ilfeld and generic abduction brace among the static splint applications. The main findings of the included articles were summarized. Conclusions: Dynamic splinting for DDH represents a valid therapeutic option in cases of instability and dislocation, especially if applied within 4–5 months of life. Dynamic splinting has a low contraindication. Static bracing is an effective option too, but only for stable hips or residual acetabular dysplasia.

Keywords: developmental dysplasia of the hip; DDH; treatment; conservative; bracing; dynamic splint; static splint

1. Introduction

Developmental dysplasia of the hip (DDH) is a common pediatric condition that has a variable incidence due to the genetic predisposition and cultural practices of different ethnicities [1]. DDH consists of a spectrum of abnormalities that range from delayed physiological development of the hip, mild capsular laxity, to acetabular deficiency, subluxation, and dislocation of the hip.

The etiology of DDH is multifactorial, involving both genetic and intrauterine factors. The gold standard for imaging infant hips is ultrasonography (US). The Graf classification system is the most adopted system for classifying infant hips basing on US images [2,3]. Radiographs may be useful starting at 4–6 months of age, but it is more suitable after femoral head ossification, which occurs by six months of age in 80% of infants [4].

The treatment of DDH has undergone significant evolution in the last few decades, depending on the patient's age and the severity of the condition. Due to abduction and

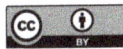

flexing of the hips while they are worn, splints and braces are applied in different diseases [5], and are actually considered the gold standard for DDH-affected children under 6 months of age with a reducible hip. The dynamic splint promotes a "dynamic reduction": the child can move his/her legs within the range permitted by the splint, maintaining the hips in flexion and abduction while restricting extension and adduction. The Pavlik harness is the most popular dynamic splint. Other dynamic splints used for treating DDH are the Tubingen splint, Frejka pillow, Von Rosen splint, Aberdeen splint, Coxaflex and Teufel brace [6–12]. The static splints promote a "rigid reduction". They consist of a metallic or hard plastic support that keeps the legs of the child in a fixed position of abduction and flexion, without the possibility of hip motion. They seem to have a higher rate of complications compared with avascular necrosis (AVN); therefore, they are less commonly used [13]. The most common static harnesses are the rhino brace, Denis Browne bar, Milgram brace and the Ilfeld harness. Generally, a dynamic splint is indicated for a reducible hip in patients that are not yet able to stand. The most accepted indication is an unstable hip that can be centered without the need for a spica cast [14]. On the other hand, static splints are an effective alternative to the dynamic splints for children more than 6–9 months of age who require continued abduction positioning because of acetabular dysplasia and/or subluxation [15].

All of the treatments with splints have risks of avascular necrosis (AVN) and femoral nerve palsy [16,17]. Higher rates of AVN are reported after unsuccessful hip reduction, presentation beyond 3 months of age, fixed dislocation and bilateral hip involvement [18–21]. The "Pavlik harness disease" is a complication following an inappropriate continuation of the harness with a dislocated hip. Femoral nerve palsy occurs on the involved side in 2.5% of patients treated with a dynamic splint, usually in the first week of treatment, and resolves within two weeks. This complication was shown to be strongly predictive of treatment failure [16].

There are few data in the literature regarding the differences between dynamic and static splints and the different varieties of each type. The aim of this study is to clarify the differences between the success, failure and complications rates of several braces available for the treatment of DDH.

2. Materials and Methods

2.1. Study Selection

According to the guidelines of the Preferred Reporting Items for Systematic Reviews and Meta-Analyses (PRISMA) [22], a systematic review of PubMed and Science Direct databases was performed by two independent authors (C.d.C. and A.V.) using the keywords "developmental dysplasia hip", "brace", "harness", "splint", and "abduction brace". Previous keywords or MeSH terms were combined in order to achieve the maximum research efficacy.

From each included article, a standard data entry form was utilized to extract the number of patients, number of hips treated, affected side, sex, age of patient at start of treatment, type of DDH, duration of splinting, number of successes and failures, success and failure according to the grade of DDH, complication rate and complication type, follow-up and period of the study.

The risk of bias assessment was performed by two independent reviewers (C.d.C. and A.V.) using the Dutch checklist form for prognosis recommended by the Cochrane Collaboration. The checklist was applied with modifications to the items that were relevant to the current study's objectives [22]. Conflicts were resolved by consultation with a senior surgeon (V.P.). Table 1 represents the risk of bias summary including the checklist items. Items could be scored as 'low risk' (+), 'high risk' (−), or 'unclear' (?). The forms were then compared and discussed to achieve a final consensus (Table 1).

Table 1. Risk of bias of the included studies.

Ref	Author	No Participant Selection Took Place	Groups Are Comparable Regarding Age	Validated Measuring System Used	Independent (Blind) Determination of Outcomes	Clear Description of Groups Available
[23]	Atalar H. et al. (2014)	+	+	+	?	+
[24]	Atan D et al. (1993)	+	?	−	?	+
[12]	Azzoni et al. (2011)	+	?	+	+	−
[25]	Cashman et al. (2002)	+	?	+	?	+
[26]	Czubak et al. (2004)	?	+	+	?	−
[27]	Eberle et al. 2003	+	?	−	?	+
[28]	Grill et al. (1988)	−	+	+	?	+
[29]	Hedequist et al. (2003)	+	−	+	?	+
[11]	Hilderaker et al. (1992)	+	+	+	?	+
[30]	Ibrahim et al. (2013)	+	?	+	?	+
[9]	Kubo et al. (2018)	+	+	−	?	+
[18]	Kitoh et al. (2009)	+	?	+	+	+
[31]	Novais et al. (2016)	+	?	+	?	+
[32]	Pavone et al. (2015)	+	?	+	?	+
[33]	Sankar et al. (2015)	+	+	+	?	+
[34]	Tegnander et al. (2001)	+	?	−	?	+
[35]	Wahlen et al. (2015)	+	+	+	?	+
[36]	Wilkinson et al. (2002)	−	?	+	?	+
[37]	Williams et al. (1999)	+	?	+	?	+

+: low risk; −: high risk; ?: unclear.

2.2. Inclusion and Exclusion Criteria

Eligible studies for the present systematic review included DDH treatment and splintage. The initial titles and abstracts screening was performed using the following inclusion criteria: treatment consisted of hip bracing without operative treatment or cast application in children aged under one-year, with a minimum average of four-months follow-up. The exclusion criteria were groups of patients with secondary hip dysplasia, including syndromic and teratogenic DDH, hip surgery treatment and casting. We also excluded all remaining duplicates, articles dealing with other topics, those with poor scientific methodology or those without an accessible abstract. Reference lists were also hand-searched for further relevant studies. Abstracts, case reports, conference presentations, editorials and expert opinions were excluded.

Two classification systems were considered: the Graf system based on US and a clinical classification according to hip stability, identifying a hip as stable, dislocatable (Barlow positive), reducible (femoral head dislocated but reducible by the Ortolani maneuver) and irreducible. For those studies that did not differentiate the subtypes of Type II into groups A, B, C and D, we considered all type II hips as type IIB in order to standardize the sample. Similar to what Grill did for his study [28], for evaluation reasons, we merged hips of grade Tönnis 1 with the type Graf IIb, grade Tönnis 2 with type Graf III, and Tönnis 3 and 4 with type Graf IV. This correlation made it possible to evaluate the material in one block. For the articles where the total number of hips was not specified, we considered the number of children to represent the number of hips.

2.3. Definition of Outcomes

We considered success to be treatment resulting in the regression of the dysplasia with recovery of the hip. In the case of hips that were irreducible, unstable at rest or on stress exam, not improved at follow-up, or when the infants underwent splinting or bracing change, spica cast application or surgical management, the treatment was assessed as "unsuccessful". On the other hand, progression of dysplasia within the first 4–8 weeks and the need for further and more invasive treatments, including casting in general anesthesia, were considered as failure. We considered only major complications that included AVN and femoral nerve palsy or other nerve palsies.

2.4. Statistical Analysis

Review Manager 5.4.1 (Review Manager (RevMan), The Cochrane Collaboration, 2020) was used to perform the meta-analysis of the selected articles that applied comparable records descriptions and had similar study cohorts. Odd ratios were combined, using the generic inverse variance. The fixed-effects model was used for all meta-analysis.

3. Results

A total of $n = 1411$ articles were found, including three articles added after the reference list analysis. After the exclusion of duplicates, $n = 367$ articles were selected. At the end of the first screening, following the previously described selection criteria, we selected $n = 29$ articles for full-text reading. Ultimately, after reading the full texts and checking the reference lists, we selected $n = 19$ articles following the previously written criteria. In Table 2 the main findings are reported according to principal author and brace/splint.

A PRISMA [21] flowchart of the method of selection and screening is provided (Figure 1).

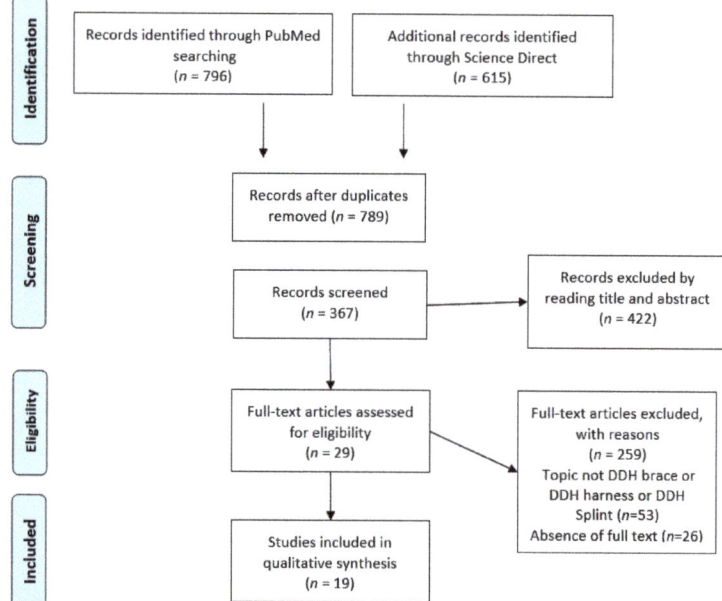

Figure 1. PRISMA (Preferred Reporting Items for Systematic Reviews and Meta-Analysis) flowchart of the systematic literature review.

In these 19 studies, a total of 5100 patients and 6755 hips were identified. Overall, a success with splintage was observed in 6272 hips with a total success rate of 93%. Fourteen studies concerned dynamic splints (74%) (dynamic splint group), and five studies were about static braces (26%) (static brace group).

Table 2. Main findings of the included studies (No. = number; f = female; m = male; ? = unknown; AVN = avascular necrosis).

Ref	Author	Brace	No. of Patients (Females, Males)	No. of Hips	Mean Age of the Brace at Treatment Onset (Weeks)	Follow Up (Months)	Success Event (%)	Complications Event (%)	AVN
[23]	Atalar et al. (2014)	Tubingen splint	49 (45 f, 4 m)	60	18	24	56 (93.3)	0 (0)	0 (0)
[24]	Atan et al. (1993)	Frejka pillow	70 (54 f, 16 m)	84	0.7	?	76 (90.5)	6 (7)	6 (7)
[24]	Atan et al. (1993)	Pavlik harness	40 (29 f, 11 m)	48	1.4	?	42 (87.5)	3 (6)	3 (6)
[12]	Azzoni et al. (2011)	Teuffel	?	59	6.1	?	59 (100)	0 (0)	0 (0)
[12]	Azzoni et al. (2011)	Coxaflex	?	59	6.1	?	58 (98.3)	0 (0)	0 (0)
[25]	Cashman et al. (2002)	Pavlik harness	332 (275 f, 57 m)	546	?	?	528 (96.7)	4 (1)	4 (1)
[26]	Czubak et al. (2004)	Pavlik harness	95 (84 f; 11 m)	?	11.5	?	90 (95)	7 (7)	7 (7)
[26]	Czubak et al. (2004)	Frejka splint	143 (129 f; 14 m)	?	11.5	?	127 (89)	17 (12)	17 (12)
[27]	Eberle et al. (2003)	Abduction brace	113	139	?	40	137 (99)	0 (0)	0 (0)
[28]	Grill et al. (1988)	Pavlik harness	2636 (2343 f; 293 m)	3611	5	53.5	3324 (92.1)	75 (2)	75 (2)
[29]	Hedequist et al. (2003)	Abduction brace	?	14	3.7	12	11 (79)	2 (14)	1 (7)
[11]	Hilderaker et al. (1992)	Frejka pillow	101	?	?	?	97 (96)	0 (0)	0 (0)
[11]	Hilderaker et al. (1992)	Von Rosen	307	?	?	?	307 (100)	0 (0)	0 (0)
[30]	Ibrahim et al. (2013)	Abduction brace	7 (7 f; 0 m)	7	10.9	33.6	6 (86)	1 (14)	1 (14)
[9]	Kubo et al. (2018)	Tubingen splint	79 (74 f; 5 m)	109	3.1	24	104 (95.4)	0 (0)	0 (0)
[18]	Kitoh et al. (2009)	Pavlik harness	210 (190 f; 20 m)	221	15.6	12	181 (81.9)	16 (7)	16 (7)
[31]	Novais et al. (2016)	Pavlik harness	135 (107 f; 28 f)	215	4.3	4	185 (86.0)	4 (2)	0 (0)
[32]	Pavone et al. (2015)	Tubingen splint	351 (248 f, 103)	544	9.7	76.8	535 (98.3)	3 (0.6)	3 (0.6)
[33]	Sankar et al. (2015)	Ilfeld	19	28	4.6	12	23 (82.1)	0 (0)	0 (0)
[34]	Tegnander et al. (2001)	Frejka pillow	108	?	16	?	105 (97.2)	1 (0.9)	1 (0.9)
[35]	Wahlen et al. (2015)	Lausanne brace (rhino-style)	33	40	11	40	35 (87.5)	0 (0)	0 (0)
[36]	Wilkinson et al. (2002)	Craig	22	28	5.3	?	24 (85.7)	0 (0)	0 (0)
[36]	Wilkinson et al. (2002)	Pavlik harness	30	43	7	?	30 (69.3)	0 (0)	0 (0)
[36]	Wilkinson et al. (2002)	Von Rosen	16	26	3.7	?	26 (100)	0 (0)	0 (0)
[37]	Williams et al. (1999)	Aberdeen Splint	86	120	?	108	118 (98.3)	2 (2)	2 (2)

The included articles [9–37] mainly focus on Pavlik harness, Frejka, and Tubingen among the dynamic splints, while the rhino-style brace, Ilfeld and generic abduction brace were considered among the static splints. The main findings of the included articles are summarized in Tables 3 and 4.

Table 3. Number of samples collected for each type of dynamic splint.

Type of Dynamic Splint	Number of Hips	Proportion within Dynamic Group
Pavlik	4779	73.2%
Tubingen	713	14.9%
Frejka pillow	436	9.1%
Von Rosen	333	5.1%
Aberdeen	120	1.8%
Coxaflex	59	0.9%
Teufel	59	0.9%
Craig	28	0.4%
TOTAL	6527	

Table 4. Number of sample collected for each type of static brace.

Type of Static Brace	Number of Hips	Proportion within Static Group
Abduction brace	160	70.2%
Rhino	40	17.5%
Ilfeld	28	12.3%
TOTAL	228	

Overall, a success with splintage was observed in 5515 hips with a total success rate of 93%. Considering only the dynamic splint group, treatment success was reached in 5287 hips with a rate of 91.3%, while a failure occurred in 427 hips with a failure rate of 8.7% (Table 4). The static brace group had a success rate of 93.0% with 212 hips healed, and a failure rate of 7.0% with 16 hips failed (Figure 2). According to the success rate, no statistically significant difference was noted between dynamic and static splinting/bracing ($p = 0.63$).

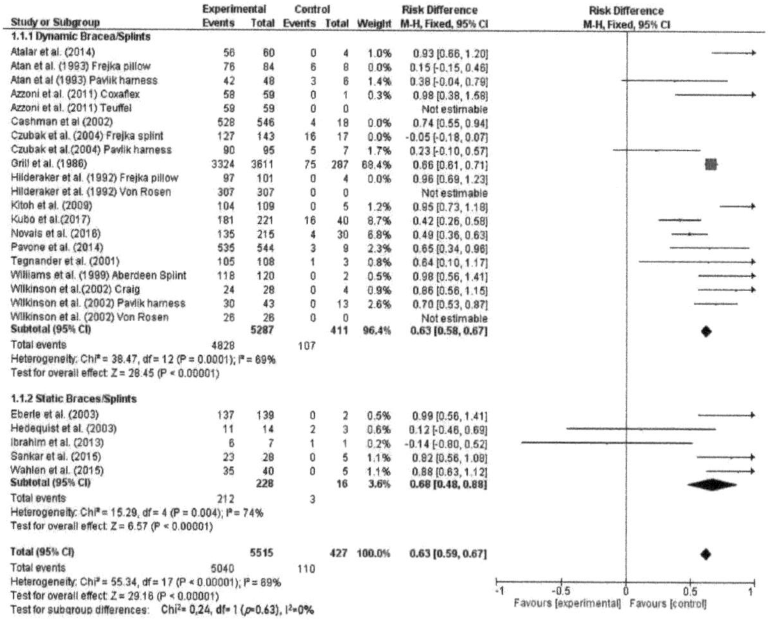

Figure 2. Forest plot of comparison: dynamic vs. static bracing/splinting. M-H = Mantel-Haenszel method; CI = confidence interval; arrow = overall effect, square = point estimate and confidence intervals of study; diamond = point estimate and confidence intervals for type of brace/splint.

Overall, the average follow-up of the studies was 36.4 months (range 2–168). The average age of patients at the start of the treatment was 6.8 weeks for the dynamic splint group (range 0.1–40) and 7.5 weeks for the patients treated with the static brace (range 1–19 weeks). The average full-time duration of splinting was 16.4 weeks (range 5–25.2) for dynamic splinting and 8.9 weeks (range 0.5–32) for the static group. Only four studies (21%) reported part-time wearing of the brace (only night-time wearing) for a mean of 10.4 weeks (range 6–16.4). Globally, a major complication occurred in 141 of the 6755 hips treated, with a rate of 2%. 136 were AVN (2%), four femoral nerve palsy (0.05%) and one growth arrest line (0.01%) over the whole sample. Among the dynamic splint group, the rate of complication was 2.1% with a total of 138 cases. The AVN rate was 2% with 134 cases. Regarding the static brace group, a complication was observed in three cases (1.3%), and two of them were AVN (AVN rate 0.8%) (Table 5).

Table 5. Complications and AVN.

	Dynamic Splint Group	Static Brace Group	Total
Complication (No. of hips)	138	3	141
Complication rate	2.1%	1.3%	2%
AVN (No. of hips)	134	2	136
AVN rate	2%	0.8%	2%

No. = number; AVN = avascular necrosis.

3.1. Abduction Brace

160 hips treated with an abduction brace were described in three different studies: Eberle et al. [27] reported that 137 of 139 hips were successfully treated, Hedequist et al. [29] found 14% (two cases) with complications including one AVN and Ibrahim et al. [30] reported only one AVN case.

3.2. Aberdeen Splint

Only one study reported DDH treatment with an Aberdeen splint [37]: Williams et al. in 1999 reported a 120-patient sample with a 98.3% success rate and a 2% rate of complications.

3.3. Coxaflex splint

Azzoni et al. (2011) [12], in a comparison study, reported 58 out of 59 successfully treated hips (98.3%), and no complications were observed in the sample.

3.4. Craig Splint

Wilkinson et al. in 2002 [36] reported the only Craig splint study that was included in the systematic review. They investigated 22 patients (28 DDH hips) and reported a 85.7% success rate with no complications.

3.5. Frejka pillow

A success rate between 89% [26] and 97.2% [34] and a complication rate between 0.9% and 12%, AVN in every case, were reported in four studies [11,24,26,34] investigating DDH patient treatment with the Frejka pillow.

3.6. Ilfeld Splint

Sankar et al. (2015) [33] evaluated 28 hips, reporting 82.1% successful treatments and no complications.

3.7. Pavlik harness

The Pavlik harness is the most represented splint with seven studies [18,24–26,28,31,36] included. These comprised a sample of 4779 hips with a success rate of 91.6%, a complication rate of 2.3% and a total of 105 AVN cases. Grill et al. [28] in 1988 described 3611 hips treated with the Pavlik harness and reported only a 7.9% rate of failure. Novais et al. [31] is the only selected study that reported four femoral nerve paralysis cases.

3.8. Rhino-Style Splint

Wahlen et al. [35], the only rhino-style splint study included in the systematic review, investigated 40 hips (33 patients) and reported a success rate of 87.5% and no complications.

3.9. Teuffel Splint

Azzoni et al. [12], in a comparison study, reported that all 59 hip treatments were successful and that no complications were observed in the sample.

3.10. Tubingen Splint

Three studies [9,23,32] investigated DDH patients treated with Tubigen splint, the largest sample after Pavlik brace (713 hips), and reported a success rate of 97.5% and a complication rate of 0.4%.

3.11. Von Rosen Splint

A 100% success rate is described for Von Rosen in 333 patients. Both Hilderaker et al. [11] and Wilkinson et al. [36] did not report complications.

4. Discussion

This analysis of DDH 6755 cases from the literature is one of the first systematic reviews to compare the outcomes and complication rates of dynamic and static hip splints. A variation of treatment timing, modalities and splints were described among the orthopedics. Dynamic splints are currently the preferred choice. According to a recent study, the type of brace that is most widely used is the Pavlik harness, accounting for 70–90% of Pediatric Orthopaedic Society of North America (POSNA) and European Paediatric Orthopaedic Society (EPOS) members, while rigid braces are chosen only in 20%, the Frejka pillow in 13% and the Von Rosen splint in less than 10% [6].

The success rate of the Pavlik harness was found to be 91.1%. Few studies have reported the efficacy of different splints: some compared the use of the Frejka pillow with the Von Rosen splint, and others described the Craig and the Von Rosen splints to be slightly superior to the Pavlik harness [27,38,39]. Surely, the Pavlik harness remains the most preferred treatment for the majority of children younger than 6 months, as it is the most thoroughly described and analyzed and found to be safe and highly effective with large samples [10,23]. The most satisfying outcomes were described with the use of Tubingen (97.5%), Von Rosen (100%), Aberdeen (98.3%%), Coxaflex (98.3%%) and Teufel (100%) splints, but the small sample of the latter three braces does not aid comparison. An increase in successful outcomes of the static braces was observed over the last few years, but only five studies for a total of 228 hips were included in the study. This may be attributable to improvements in the achievement of custom-made braces over time and to more numerous cases of low- and mid-grade of dysplasia being encountered. A good advantage is that the design avoids any maladjustment for the user, unlike Pavlik's harness, so that the brace is easily applied without any risk of improper positioning; moreover, static braces should be also used in children older than 6 months [35].

We found a success rate of the static brace group of 93.0% and a failure rate of 7.0%. Even if the number of total cases included is only 212 hips, the static brace seems to be effective. Several authors reported series of patients in whom static bracing successfully stabilized persistent posterior dislocations following Pavlik harness failure [27,29,33,40], and in three of these studies [27,29,30], the static brace was applied after Pavlik treatment failure, causing a decrease in the percentage of success. In fact, there were a total of 49 hips with a success rate of 69.3%, but with a much higher rate of failure concerning irreducible and dislocatable but reducible hips.

Static bracing has been previously described as a viable option for treating DDH after a Pavlik failure and has the obvious advantages of avoiding both general anesthesia and a spica cast, which expose the child to several risks [41]. Eighty-two percent of hips that fail using the Pavlik harness respond successfully to rigid hip abduction bracing, but if rigid bracing cannot reduce the hip at the beginning of treatment, it should be avoided [27,31]. On the other hand, Ibrahim et al. [30] demonstrated opposite results, with a 100% of failure over seven hips, finding no advantage of static splinting but only an unnecessary delay of the time to closed reduction. However, it should be noticed that three patients had irreducible hips. Observing these series, even after an initial failure of dynamic splint treatment, an attempt of treatment with a static brace should be done for 3–4 weeks, but in our opinion, the condition is that the hip must be well located in the acetabulum. However, this switch is generally preferred by American surgeons and poorly performed by European physicians [6,29]. The mechanism by which a static splint may succeed where the Pavlik harness failed is unclear. The most probable reason may be related to inferior dislocation aggravated by flexion. A rigid or semirigid brace generally holds hips in less flexion than a standard Pavlik harness fitting and may be useful for certain dislocations that are predominantly inferior. The rigidity of the device may provide more structure for certain hips that remain excessively lax even within a Pavlik harness. It may also be that rigid orthoses make it easier to apply for certain families [29,42].

Even though dynamic splints observe the safe position suggested by Ramsey [43], spontaneous AVN remans the main complication in dysplastic hip treatment and must be considered as iatrogenic secondary to splintage [44]. Several studies report the AVN rate as negligible when the splints straps are properly adjusted [18,43,45]. The complication rate of the Pavlik harness in these series is 2.3% with an AVN rate of 2.2%. The Frejka pillow has the highest AVN rate, with 5.6% of 436 hips, due to the extreme abduction of this splint. Even if this review reports high rates of success and few complications for the Von Rosen splint, one should be considerate of the small sample. Also, the degrees of abduction seem to be too extreme for a safe treatment. Even if several studies found an increased risk of AVN with more rigid braces, we found an AVN rate of 0.8%, and if we do not consider the irreducible hips, the value decrease further. Static splints should be used only if the epiphysis is well positioned in the acetabular base, because this type of brace can often fail to center the hip in the acetabulum, and especially because a not-well-centered epiphysis will be strongly stressed against the superior roof of the acetabulum by a rigid splint, damaging the cartilaginous component and delaying healing, with the possibility of worsening the dislocation [13]. We did not find a correlation between AVN rate and duration of treatment. The treatment of residual acetabular dysplasia in children older than six months remains challenging. Spontaneous resolution of this residual dysplasia without intervention is unlikely in children over six months of age [46]. Some studies support the use of static splints to treat residual acetabular dysplasia in older infants when they have outgrown the Pavlik harness, improving the acetabular index, but the data are still limited [39,47,48]. However, a part-time rigid abduction brace is often used at many centers to produce some improvement in the acetabular index without a major impact on the child's activity, but the optimal duration of the brace is still unclear [39].

An important limit is the improper positioning of the brace, which is often an iatrogenic cause of damage. Insufficient hip flexion is one of the most common pitfalls that can lead to an insufficient reduction. In dynamic braces/splints, another risk is that the distal components can be positioned too distally at the level of the knee. The incorrect position of the distal part of brace could cause a limited hip reductive effect in the acetabulum due to a lever mechanism [13]. A cause of failure is also parents' low cooperation with the use of the brace. Parents play a key role in the effective use of the splint, and they must be educated about the proper use of the harness to increase the chance of success [14]. Regarding the approach of application of the splint, the recent survey of EPOS and POSNA members found that around 20% of surgeons allowed their patients to always wear clothes underneath their brace, 15% never allowed clothes, 20% only allowed clothes once the hip was clinically stable, and about 22% only allowed underwear [6].

This study has several limitations, including the sample heterogeneity for number, age of population and grade of dysplasia and the bias risk related to no common definition of successful outcome. Larger samples, comparative studies and defined quality standards are needed, especially for the static braces. The classification system of the grade of DDH is not homogeneous in all the articles included; therefore, there exists bias in the analysis. Several studies have short-term follow-ups that cannot accurately verify the success of the treatment and the presence of a delayed AVN.

5. Conclusions

Dynamic splinting for DDH represents a valid therapeutic option in cases of instability and dislocation, especially if applied within 4–5 months of life. Dynamic splinting has a low contraindication and is very well tolerated. The Pavlik harness is still the most used brace, but the Tubingen splint showed better outcomes with major tolerance and compliance. The limits concern the accurate indications and timing of initiation. The static brace is an effective option too, but only for stable hips: it is imperative that the femoral head be well centered in the acetabular base for a safe treatment. Static braces can be also useful in cases of residual acetabular dysplasia.

Author Contributions: Conceptualization, C.d.C. and G.T.; methodology, M.S.; software, A.V.; validation, V.P., and P.P.; formal analysis, L.L.; investigation, C.d.C.; resources, A.V.; data curation, M.S.; writing—original draft preparation, A.V.; writing—review and editing, G.T.; visualization, G.S.; supervision, V.P.; project administration, V.P.; funding acquisition, V.P. All authors have read and agreed to the published version of the manuscript.

Funding: This research received no external funding.

Institutional Review Board Statement: Not applicable.

Informed Consent Statement: Not applicable.

Data Availability Statement: No new data were created or analyzed in this study. Data sharing is not applicable to this article.

Acknowledgments: Thanks for funding "Open Access" to PIA.CE.RI. of University of Catania.

Conflicts of Interest: The authors declare no conflict of interest.

References

1. Loder, R.T.; Skopelja, E.N. The epidemiology and demographics of hip dysplasia. *ISRN Orthop.* **2011**, *2011*, 238607. [CrossRef]
2. Graf, R. The diagnosis of congenital hip-joint dislocation by the ultrasonic Combound treatment. *Arch. Orthop. Trauma. Surg.* **1980**, *97*, 117–133. [CrossRef] [PubMed]
3. Graf, R. *Hip Sonography: Diagnosis and Management of Infant Hip Dysplasia*, 2nd ed.; Springer: Berlin/Heidelberg, Germany, 2006; pp. 1–114.
4. Shaw, B.A.; Segal, L.S. Section on Orthopaedics. Evaluation and referral for developmental dysplasia of the hip in infants. *Pediatrics* **2016**, *138*, e20163107. [CrossRef] [PubMed]
5. Pavone, V.; Vescio, A.; Montemagno, M.; de Cristo, C.; Lucenti, L.; Pavone, P.; Testa, G. Perinatal Femoral Fracture: A Ten-Year Observational Case Series Study. *Children* **2020**, *7*, 156. [CrossRef]
6. Alves, C.; Truong, W.H.; Thompson, M.V.; Suryavanshi, J.R.; Penny, C.L.; Do, H.T.; Dodwell, E.R. Diagnostic and treatment preferences for developmental dysplasia of the hip: A survey of EPOS and POSNA members. *J. Child. Orthop.* **2018**, *12*, 236–244. [CrossRef] [PubMed]
7. Gulati, V.; Eseonu, K.; Sayani, J.; Ismail, N.; Uzoigwe, C.; Choudhury, M.Z.; Gulati, P.; Aqil, A.; Tibrewal, S. Developmental dysplasia of the hip in the newborn: A systematic review. *World J. Orthop.* **2013**, *4*, 32–41. [CrossRef]
8. Bernau, A. Die Tübinger Hüftbeugeschiene zur Behandlung der Hüftdysplasie. *Z. Orthop.* **1990**, *128*, 432–435. [CrossRef] [PubMed]
9. Kubo, H.; Pilge, H.; Weimann-Stahlschmidt, K.; Stefanovska, K.; Westhoff, B.; Krauspe, R. Use of the Tübingen splint for the initial management of severely dysplastic and unstable hips in newborns with DDH: An alternative to Fettweis plaster and Pavlik harness. *Arch. Orthop. Trauma Surg.* **2018**, *138*, 149–153. [CrossRef]

10. Dwan, K.; Kirkham, J.; Paton, R.W.; Morley, E.; Newton, A.W.; Perry, D.C. Splinting for the non-operative management of developmental dysplasia of the hip (DDH) in children under six months of age. *Coch. Data. Syst. Rev.* **2017**, *7*, CD012717. [CrossRef]
11. Hinderaker, T.; Rygh, M.; Udén, A. The von Rosen splint compared with the Frejka pillow: A study of 408 neonatally unstable hips. *Acta. Orthop. Scand.* **1992**, *63*, 389–392. [CrossRef]
12. Azzoni, R.; Cabitza, P. A comparative study on the effectiveness of two different devices in the management of developmental dysplasia of the hip in infants. *Min. Ped.* **2011**, *63*, 355–361.
13. Pagnotta, G.; Ruzzini, L.; Oggiano, L. Dynamic management of developmental dysplasia of the hip. *Arch. Ortop. Reumatol.* **2012**, *123*, 21–22. [CrossRef]
14. Mubarak, S.; Garfin, S.; Vance, R.; McKinnon, B.; Sutherland, D. Pitfalls in the use of the Pavlik harness for treatment of congenital dysplasia, subluxation, and dislocation of the hip. *J. Bone Jt. Surg. Am.* **1981**, *63*, 1239–1248. [CrossRef] [PubMed]
15. Weinstein, S.L.; Mubarak, S.J.; Wenger, D.R. Developmental hip dysplasia and dislocation: Part II. *Instr. Course Lect.* **2004**, *53*, 531–542. [CrossRef]
16. Murnaghan, M.L.; Browne, R.H.; Sucato, D.J.; Birch, J. Femoral nerve palsy in Pavlik harness treatment for developmental dysplasia of the hip. *J. Bone Jt. Surg. Am.* **2011**, *93*, 493–499. [CrossRef]
17. Pollet, V.; Pruijs, H.; Sakkers, R.; Castelein, R. Results of Pavlik harness treatment in children with dislocated hips between the age of six and twenty-four months. *J. Pediatr. Orthop.* **2010**, *30*, 437–442. [CrossRef]
18. Kitoh, H.; Kawasumi, M.; Ishiguro, N. Predictive factors for unsuccessful treatment of developmental dysplasia of the hip by the Pavlik harness. *J. Pediatr. Orthop.* **2009**, *29*, 552–557. [CrossRef]
19. Suzuki, S.; Yamamuro, T. Avascular necrosis in patients treated with the Pavlik harness for congenital dislocation of the hip. *J. Bone Jt. Surg. Am.* **1990**, *72*, 1048–1055. [CrossRef]
20. Inoue, T.; Naito, M.; Nomiyama, H. Treatment of developmental dysplasia of the hp with the Pavlik harness: Factors for predicting unsuccessful reduction. *J. Pediatr. Orthop. B* **2001**, *10*, 186–191.
21. Lerman, J.A.; Emans, J.B.; Millis, M.B.; Share, J.; Zurakowski, D.; Kasser, J.R. Early failure of Pavlik harness treatment for developmental hip dysplasia: Clinical and ultrasound predictors. *J. Pediatr. Orthop.* **2001**, *21*, 348–353. [CrossRef] [PubMed]
22. Moher, D.; Liberati, A.; Tetzlaff, J.; Altman, D.G.; PRISMA Group. Preferred Reporting Items for Systematic Reviews and Meta-Analyses: The PRISMA Statement. *PLoS Med.* **2009**, *6*, e1000097. [CrossRef]
23. Atalar, H.; Gunay, C.; Komurcu, M. Functional treatment of developmental hip dysplasia with the Tübingen hip flexion splint. *Hip Int.* **2014**, *24*, 295–301. [CrossRef]
24. Atar, D.; Lehman, W.B.; Tenenbaum, Y.; Grant, A.D. Pavlik harnes versus Frejka splint in treatment of developmental dysplasia of the hip: Bicenter study. *J. Pediatr. Orthop.* **1993**, *13*, 311–313. [CrossRef]
25. Cashman, J.P.; Round, J.; Taylor, G.; Clarke, N.M. The natural history of developmental dysplasia of the hip after early supervised treatment in the Pavlik harness. A prospective, longitudinal follow-up. *J. Bone Jt. Surg. Br.* **2002**, *84*, 418–425. [CrossRef]
26. Czubak, J.; Piontek, T.; Niciejewski, K.; Magnowski, P.; Majek, M.; Płończak, M. Retrospective analysis of the non-surgical treatment of developmental dysplasia of the hip using Pavlik harness and Frejka pillow: Comparison of both methods. *Ortop. Traumatol. Rehabil.* **2004**, *6*, 9–13.
27. Eberle, C.F. Plastazote abduction orthosis in the management of neonatal hip instability. *J. Pediatr. Orthop.* **2003**, *23*, 607–616. [CrossRef] [PubMed]
28. Grill, F.; Bensahel, H.; Canadell, J.; Dungl, P.; Matasovic, T.; Vizkelety, T. The Pavlik harness in the treatment of congenital dislocating hip: Report on a multicenter study of the European Paediatric Orthopaedic Society. *J. Pediatr. Orthop.* **1988**, *8*, 1–8. [CrossRef]
29. Hedequist, D.; Kasser, J.; Emans, J. Use of an abduction brace for developmental dysplasia of the hip after failure of Pavlik harness use. *J. Pediatr. Orthop.* **2003**, *23*, 175–177. [CrossRef]
30. Ibrahim, D.A.; Skaggs, D.L.; Choi, P.D. Abduction bracing after Pavlik harness failure: An effective alternative to closed reduction and spica casting? *J. Pediatr. Orthop.* **2013**, *33*, 536–539. [CrossRef] [PubMed]
31. Novais, E.N.; Kestel, L.A.; Carry, P.M.; Meyers, M.L. Higher Pavlik harness treatment failure is seen in Graf type IV ortolani-positive hips in males. *Clin. Orthop. Relat. Res.* **2016**, *474*, 1847–1854. [CrossRef]
32. Pavone, V.; Testa, G.; Riccioli, M.; Evola, F.R.; Avondo, S.; Sessa, G. Treatment of developmental dysplasia of hip with Tubingen hip flexion splint. *J. Pediatr. Orthop.* **2015**, *35*, 485–489. [CrossRef] [PubMed]
33. Sankar, W.N.; Nduaguba, A.; Flynn, J.M. Ilfeld abduction orthosis is an effective second-line treatment after failure of Pavlik harness for infants with developmental dysplasia of the hip. *J. Bone Jt. Surg. Am.* **2015**, *97*, 292–297. [CrossRef] [PubMed]
34. Tegnander, A.; Holen, K.J.; Anda, S.; Terjesen, T. Good results after treatment with the Frejka pillow for hip dysplasia in newborns: A 3-year to 6-year follow-up study. *J. Pediatr. Orthop. B* **2001**, *10*, 173–179. [PubMed]
35. Wahlen, R.; Zambelli, P. Treatment of the developmental dysplasia of the hip with an abduction brace in children up to 6 months old. *Adv. Orthop.* **2015**, *2015*, 103580. [CrossRef]
36. Wilkinson, A.G.; Sherlock, D.A.; Murray, G.D. The efficacy of the Pavlik harness, the Craig splint and the von Rosen splint in the management of neonatal dysplasia of the hip: A comparative study. *J. Bone Jt. Surg. Br.* **2002**, *84*, 716–719. [CrossRef]
37. Williams, P.R.; Jones, D.A.; Bishay, M. Avascular necrosis and the Aberdeen splint in developmental dysplasia of the hip. *J. Bone Jt. Surg. Br.* **1999**, *81*, 1023–1028. [CrossRef]

38. Noordin, S.; Umer, M.; Hafeez, K.; Nawaz, H. Developmental dysplasia of the hip. *Orthop. Rev. (Pavia)* **2010**, *2*, e19. [CrossRef]
39. Gans, I.; Flynn, J.M.; Sankar, W.N. Abduction bracing for residual acetabular dysplasia in infantile DDH. *J. Pediatr. Orthop.* **2013**, *33*, 714–718. [CrossRef]
40. Swaroop, V.T.; Mubarak, S.J. Difficult-to-treat Ortolani-positive hip: Improved success with new treatment protocol. *J. Pediatr. Orthop.* **2009**, *29*, 224–230. [CrossRef] [PubMed]
41. Olsen, E.A.; Brambrink, A.M. Anesthesia for the young child undergoing ambulatory procedures: Current concerns regarding harm to the developing brain. *Curr. Opin. Anaesthesiol.* **2013**, *26*, 677–684. [CrossRef]
42. Viere, R.G.; Birch, J.G.; Herring, J.A. Use of the Pavlik harness in congenital dislocation of the hip: An analysis of failures of treatment. *J. Bone Jt. Surg. Am.* **1990**, *72*, 238–244. [CrossRef]
43. Ramsey, P.L.; Lasser, S.; MacEwen, G.D. Congenital dislocation of the hip. Use of the Pavlik harness in the child during the first six months of life. *J. Bone Jt. Surg. Am.* **1976**, *58*, 1000–1004. [CrossRef]
44. Gage, J.R.; Winter, R.B. Avascular necrosis of the capital femoral epiphysis as a complication of closed reduction of congenital dislocation of the hip: A critical review of twenty years' experience at Gillette Children's Hospital. *J. Bone Jt. Surg. Am.* **1972**, *54*, 373–388. [CrossRef]
45. Kalamchi, A.; MacFarlane, R., 3rd. The Pavlik harness: Results in patients over three months of age. *J. Pediatr. Orthop.* **1982**, *2*, 3–8. [CrossRef]
46. Vitale, M.G.; Skaggs, D.L. Developmental dysplasia of the hip from six months to four years of age. *J. Am. Acad. Orthop. Surg.* **2001**, *9*, 401–411. [CrossRef] [PubMed]
47. Fabry, G. Clinical practice: The hip from birth to adolescence. *Eur. J. Pediatr.* **2010**, *169*, 143–148. [CrossRef]
48. Harris, I.E.; Dickens, R.; Menelaus, M.B. Use of the Pavlik harness for hip displacements. When to abandon treatment. *Clin. Orthop. Relat. Res.* **1992**, *281*, 29–33.

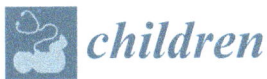

Article

The Relationship between the Dominant Hand and the Occurrence of the Supracondylar Humerus Fracture in Pediatric Orthopedics

Alexandru Herdea [1,2], Alexandru Ulici [1,2,*], Alexandra Toma [3], Bogdan Voicu [4] and Adham Charkaoui [3]

[1] Pediatric Orthopedics Department, "Grigore Alexandrescu" Children's Emergency Hospital, 011743 Bucharest, Romania; alexherdea@yahoo.com
[2] 11th Department, "Carol Davila" University of Medicine and Pharmacy, 050474 Bucharest, Romania
[3] Department of Morphological and Functional Sciences, Faculty of Medicine and Pharmacy, "Dunărea de Jos" University of Galați, 800008 Galați, Romania; dr.alexandratoma@gmail.com (A.T.); charkaoui.adham@gmail.com (A.C.)
[4] General Medicine Department, "Carol Davila" University of Medicine and Pharmacy, 050474 Bucharest, Romania; bogdanvoicu413@yahoo.com
* Correspondence: alexandru.ulici@umfcd.ro; Tel.: +40-723188988

Abstract: It is known that during a fall, a child would rather protect their dominant hand by using the non-dominant one, although the role of handedness in upper limb fractures has not been studied in-depth. We carried out a retrospective, cross-sectional cohort study, including pediatric patients who presented to the emergency room with a supracondylar humerus fracture following an injury by falling from the same height. In total, 245 patients were selected and grouped according to age. In the 1–3 years group, no statistical significance was found between hand dominance and the side of fracture ($p = 0.7315$). During preschool years (4–6 years old), the non-dominant hand is more often involved ($p = 0.03$, odds ratio: 3.5). In the 7–14 years group this trend was maintained and actually increased ($p = 0.052$, odds ratio: 3.8). We might conclude that children tend to protect their dominant hand by falling on their non-dominant one. The main objective of this study is to highlight a link between handedness and the side of the body where the hand fracture will be identified in the pediatric population, regarding supracondylar humerus fracture.

Keywords: supracondylar humerus fracture; pediatric; humerus fracture; upper limb fracture; fracture laterality; handedness; pediatric orthopedics

Citation: Herdea, A.; Ulici, A.; Toma, A.; Voicu, B.; Charkaoui, A. The Relationship between the Dominant Hand and the Occurrence of the Supracondylar Humerus Fracture in Pediatric Orthopedics. *Children* **2021**, *8*, 51. https://doi.org/10.3390/children8010051

Received: 10 November 2020
Accepted: 13 January 2021
Published: 15 January 2021

Publisher's Note: MDPI stays neutral with regard to jurisdictional claims in published maps and institutional affiliations.

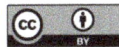

Copyright: © 2021 by the authors. Licensee MDPI, Basel, Switzerland. This article is an open access article distributed under the terms and conditions of the Creative Commons Attribution (CC BY) license (https://creativecommons.org/licenses/by/4.0/).

1. Introduction

Supracondylar humerus fracture is a common type of elbow fracture in the pediatric population [1,2]. The peak incidence occurs between five and eight years, with a medium age of six years [3]. The literature findings reveal that two thirds of elbow fractures admitted to the hospital are supracondylar humerus fractures [1,4].

Supracondylar humerus fractures can result from traumatic events that interest the upper limb during both flexion and extension of the elbow, although hyperextension mechanism is more often incriminated [5]. They usually occur during sport and leisure activities as a result of falling from the same height or from under 3 m [6].

Complications of supracondylar humerus fracture include neurovascular injuries, compartment syndrome, delay of consolidation or myositis ossificans [7].

Handedness is known to be a factor involved in orthopedic pathologies besides the one being addressed by our study. In a record review of 169 patients with carpal tunnel syndrome, Reinstein found that it occurs significantly more often in the dominant hand than in the non-dominant one [8]. Goldberg et al. studied a group of 245 girls with idiopathic scoliosis with a minimum age of eight years and concluded that the lower thoracic curvature develops with the convexity towards the dominant side in 82% of the cases, with the correlation between scoliosis configuration and handedness being statistically significant [9]. Borton et al. found on a group of 426 children with unilateral fractures of the distal forearm that the overall risk of a fracture to occur on the non-dominant side was 57% [10]. The non-dominant side may be injury-prone simply because of the dominant hand that is involved in an ongoing activity or it is used to cling to an object in an attempt to prevent the fall [11].

Although there are many studies that address the management of such fractures and the efficacy of different treatments, only a few of them analyze the link between a child's handedness and the side they are more likely to sustain a fracture [10–12].

Our study aims to highlight a link between the dominant hand and the side of a supracondylar humerus fracture in the pediatric population. The hypothesis is that children tend to guard their dominant hand in the event of a fall, thus exposing their non-dominant one to trauma because the dominant one might be involved in an activity.

2. Materials and Methods

The study took place in the Pediatric Orthopedics Department at "Grigore Alexandrescu" Children's Emergency Hospital, Bucharest, Romania, located in an urban area, between May 2019 and November 2019. The ethics committee of "Grigore Alexandrescu" Children's Emergency Clinical Hospital of Bucharest approved this study on 16 April 2019. The identification number of the study is 24/16 April 2019. An informed consent was obtained from the parents of all the participants.

We performed a retrospective, cross-sectional cohort study that began on 30 May 2019 and ended on 12 November 2019.

Our inclusion criteria comprised: positive diagnosis (clinical examination along with elbow x-rays from both frontal and lateral views), trauma history (falling from the same height during recreational activities), age, sex and hand dominance. We excluded patients that had a history of falling from a different plane, high energy trauma, road accidents, incomplete patient data and lack of informed consent. Falling from the same height was defined as falling from a standing point as a result of slipping on a surface or tripping on objects no higher than knee-level, below 1.5 m.

The following data was acquired and analyzed: age, sex, side of fracture and dominant hand. The patients were classified by age in three groups: 1–3 years old (toddlers), 4–6 years old (preschoolers), 7–14 years old (schoolers). All of the patients included in the study group sustained a supracondylar humerus fracture with the elbow in extension. The Gartland classification and information about the therapeutic conduct were available but we considered it being irrelevant to the hypothesis of the study.

For the age group of 1–3 years old, handedness was established by asking the parents which hand does the child most often put in his mouth, and which hand is used to reach for objects whether they are given to him by someone else or not. In the 4–6 years old group, they were asked which hand is most often used to eat, play or draw. In the group of schoolers 7–14 years old, we asked which hand the child used for writing or brushing their hair.

Statistical analysis of data was performed through the GraphPad prism 6.1 and Medcalc 14 programs, where we calculated the odds ratio and statistical significance using Fisher's exact test. A confidence interval of 95% was used and a $p < 0.05$ was considered statistically significant.

3. Results

A total of 403 patients presented to the emergency room in the selected time frame and were diagnosed with supracondylar humerus fracture. In total, 245 of the patients met the inclusion criteria. The remaining 158 patients were excluded due to incomplete data (49), lack of consent (35) or history of high energy trauma or road accidents (74).

Among the selected patients, 112 (45.7%) were girls, with a mean age of 5.25 years, and 133 (54.3%) were boys, with a mean age of 6 years.

The interrater reliability test that uses the dominant member as a decisional criterion and the laterality of fracture as the variability criterion demonstrates the lack of any direct, linear ($k = -0.109$) connection, thus refuting the test hypothesis of the occurrence of fractures in the dominant member. Practically, the test suggests the possibility that the fractures may appear in the non-dominant member, a hypothesis that we will test in the following research.

Following the main objective of this study, we performed a Fisher analysis that compared the frequency of fracture distribution by handedness. Thus, it can be seen in the graphical representation (Figure 1A) that patients tend to have non-dominant limb fractures ($p = 0.01$). Odds ratio analysis (OR = 2.41) can be interpreted as an independent risk factor for right-handed patients to undergo fractures on the left humerus, and for left-handed patients to undergo fractures on the right humerus.

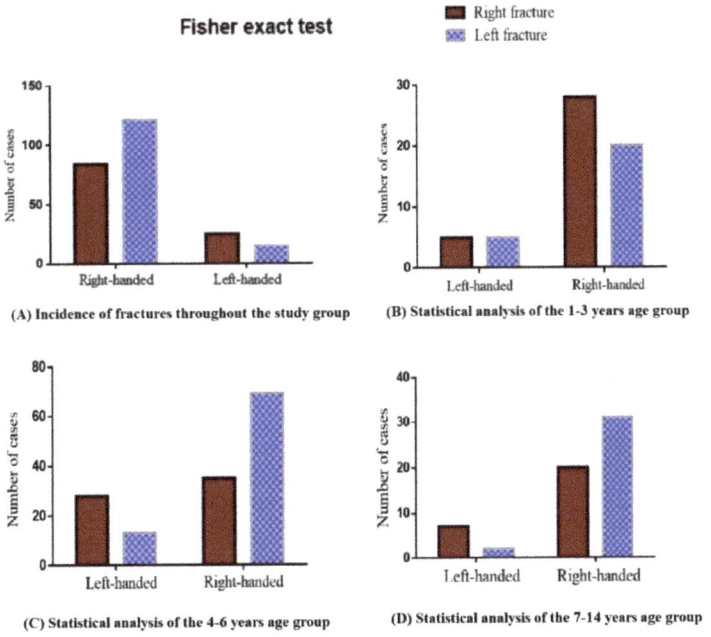

Figure 1. Results of Fischer's exact test for the entire study group (**A**) and age group 1–3 (**B**), 4–6 (**C**) and 7–14 (**D**).

There were 136 (55.5%) supracondylar fractures of the left humerus and 109 (44.5%) supracondylar fractures of the right humerus.

Fractures of the dominant hand occurred in 99 (40.4%) patients, while the rest of them sustained a fracture on the non-dominant side. Pertaining to right-handed patients, 121 (59%) of them sustained a fracture on the left side, while 84 (41%) of them had the right humerus fractured. Pertaining to left-handed patients, 15 (37.5%) of them sustained a fracture on the left side, while 25 (62.5%) of them had the right humerus fractured.

The average age of the entire study group was 5.7 years and the median was 6 years, as seen in Figure 2. Using the D'Agostino and Pearson omnibus normality test, Wilcoxon Signed Rank Test and one sample t test it was found that the highest incidence of fractures was around the age of 6 ($p < 0.0001$).

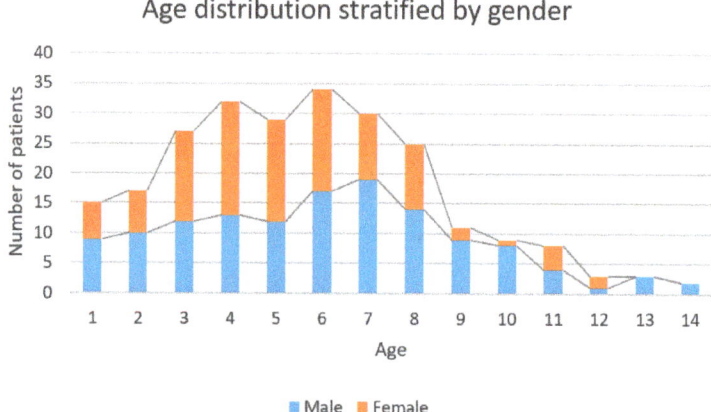

Figure 2. Age distribution stratified by gender.

In the age group of 1–3 years, there were 59 (24.1%) patients, 31 (52.5%) boys and 28 (47.5%) girls. In this group, 49 (83.1%) were right-handed children, 29 (59.2%) suffered a fracture on the right side and 20 (40.8%) on the left side. The remaining 10 (16.9%) patients were left-handed, five of them (50%) suffering a fracture on the right side and five of them (50%) on the left side. There was no statistical difference in fracture distribution among toddlers ($p = 0.7315$) pertaining to Fisher's exact test (Figure 1B).

In the age group of 4–6 years, there were 95 (38.8%) patients, 42 (44.2%) boys and 53 (55.8%) girls. In this group, 77 (81.1%) were right-handed, 28 (36.4%) underwent supracondylar humerus fracture on the right side and 49 (63.6%) suffered a fracture on the left humerus. The remaining 18 (18.9%) were left-handed, 12 (66.7%) of them being diagnosed with supracondylar fracture of the right humerus and six (33.3%) of them having the left side involved (Figure 1C). Non-dominant upper limb fractures were best represented in this group with the correlation being statistically significant ($p = 0.03$) as a result of the Fisher's exact test. The risk of non-dominant limb fracture, as calculated using the odds ratio, was 3.5 times higher than the risk of dominant hand fracture (OR = 3.5).

In the age group of 7–14 years, there were 91 (37.1%) patients, 60 (65.9%) boys and 31 (34.1%) girls, as shown in Figure 1D. There were 79 right-handed (86.8%) children, 27 (34.2%) of whom suffered a supracondylar fracture of the right humerus, the rest of the 52 patients (65.8%) having the left upper limb injured. There were 12 left-handed people (13.2%), 8 (66.7%) of whom sustained a right upper limb injury, the remaining four (33.3%) suffering a fracture of the left elbow. In this age group there is a clear tendency of fractures to occur in the non-dominant limb, but analyzing the frequency distribution using Fisher's exact test, it was not statistically significant ($p = 0.052$). The risk of non-dominant limb fracture was 3.8 higher than the risk of dominant limb fracture (OR = 3.852) in schoolers.

In order to determine an age cut-off where non-dominant limb fractures begins to predominate, we performed a ROC analysis that uses the non-dominant limb fracture as a criterion for variability and age as a variable. Thus, the ROC analysis detected a three-year cut-off point, with a sensitivity of 82.9% and a specificity of 34.3% from which patients tend to sustain non-dominant supracondylar humerus fractures. Area under the ROC curve was close to 0.5 (AUC = 0.58), but due to the large number of patients in this study it was statistically significant ($p = 0.03$). Based on this analysis the establishment of the handedness below three years of age is irrelevant to the laterality of fracture.

4. Discussion

In order to correctly assess a supracondylar humerus fracture, clinical examination and conventional x-rays are needed [13]. Thus, the confusion between a supracondylar humerus fracture and a nursemaid's elbow, another common elbow trauma in children under six, can be ruled out [14]. The treatment varies accordingly to the Gartland classification, ranging from closed reduction and casting to closed or open reduction and pinning using K wires [15]. In most severe cases, Computed Tomography followed by 3D reconstruction and 3D printing can help the orthopedic surgeon plan the safest surgery [16].

Vaquero-Picado et al. observed that this type of fracture occurs 1.5 times more often on the non-dominant limb than on the dominant one in male patients [3]. Calculating the same risk rate in our study population, we obtained a value of 2.41.

Given the relationship between the mean age of 5.7 years and the group's median age of six years, we can surely say that the peak incidence of supracondylar humerus fractures occurs at six years old. This is consistent with Vaquero-Picado et al. who found the peak incidence of supracondylar humerus fractures to occur between five and eight years old, with the mean age being six years [3].

Studying data from the age group of 1–3 years shows no statistical significance between hand dominance and the laterality of fracture. We can say that in this case, a supracondylar humerus fracture may occur randomly and this is why we cannot continue to discuss possible risks at this age.

Data obtained from older age groups sustains the hypothesis that a supracondylar humerus fracture occurs more frequently on the non-dominant hand. Preschoolers are 3.5 times more likely to fracture their non-dominant hand. In this group, the correlation is statistically significant ($p = 0.03$). Preschoolers also tend to suffer non-dominant limb fractures, although the p-value was not statistically significant ($p = 0.052$). Mortensson et al. noticed that the dominant hand might be involved in an activity during a fall and that is why the traumatic event affects mainly the non-dominant hand [12].

One of the limitations we encountered in this study relates to the group of toddlers, as hand dominance could not be firmly established by the parents in some cases. Another drawback was the lack of ambidextrous children in this study as none presented to the pediatric orthopedic emergency room during our data collection. Fracture classification and preferred treatment were not taken into account.

Our objectives were met and the hypothesis that the non-dominant hand is more frequently injured in the event of elbow trauma was confirmed. The findings of our study were consistent with those of other researchers as Hassan [11] and Borton et al. [10].

5. Conclusions

The relationship between handedness and laterality of supracondylar humerus fractures is relevant only among children older than three years of age, because hand dominance starts to be relevant after this cut-off. Before the age of three, this type of fracture occurs as a random event as no statistical correlation was found.

Considering the above, we recommend the establishment of fracture prevention techniques during a fall accident so that the forces may be evenly distributed on both limbs whenever possible, avoiding the instinctive maneuver to fall on the non-dominant limb. These could be introduced in sport-related activities, both individual and collective.

Further studies can be conducted to evaluate this correlation according to the children's activity preceding the traumatic event, as well as to monitor ambidextrous children.

Author Contributions: Conceptualization, A.U., A.H. and A.C.; methodology, A.H.; software, A.T.; validation, A.H., A.C. and A.U.; formal analysis, B.V.; investigation, B.V.; resources, A.H., A.C., A.T., B.V. and A.U.; data curation, B.V.; writing—original draft preparation, A.H.; writing—review and editing, A.C., A.T. and B.V.; visualization, A.T.; supervision, A.H., A.U. All authors have read and agreed to the published version of the manuscript.

Funding: This research received no external funding.

Institutional Review Board Statement: The study was conducted according to the guidelines of the Declaration of Helsinki, and approved by the Ethics Committee of "Grigore Alexandrescu" Children's Emergency Clinical Hospital of Bucharest, on 16 April 2019. Protocol code is 24/16 April 2019.

Informed Consent Statement: Informed consent was obtained from the parents of all subjects involved in the study.

Data Availability Statement: The data are not publicly available due to ethical reasons and patient privacy.

Conflicts of Interest: The authors declare no conflict of interest.

References

1. Omid, R.; Choi, P.; Skaggs, D. Supracondylar humeral fractures in children. *J. Bone Jt. Surg. Am.* **2008**, *90*, 1121–1132. [CrossRef] [PubMed]
2. Guo, L.; Zhang, X.-N.; Yang, J.-P.; Wang, Z.; Qi, Y.; Zhu, S.; Meng, X.-H. A systematic review and meta-analysis of two different managements for supracondylar humeral fractures in children. *J. Orthop. Surg. Res.* **2018**, *13*, 14.
3. Vaquero-Picado, A.; González-Morán, G.; Moraleda, L. Management of supracondylar fractures of the humerus in children. *EFORT Open Rev.* **2018**, *3*, 526–540. [CrossRef] [PubMed]
4. Kumar, V.; Singh, A. Fracture supracondylar humerus: A review. *J. Clin. Diagn. Res.* **2016**, *10*, RE01–RE06. [CrossRef] [PubMed]
5. Mahan, S.; May, C.; Kocher, M. Operative management of displaced flexion supracondylar humerus fractures in children. *J. Pediatric Orthop.* **2007**, *27*, 551–556. [CrossRef] [PubMed]
6. Houshian, S.; Mehdi, B.; Larsen, M. The epidemiology of elbow fracture in children: Analysis of 355 fractures, with special reference to supracondylar humerus fractures. *J. Orthop. Sci.* **2001**, *6*, 312–315. [CrossRef] [PubMed]
7. Bălănescu, R.; Ulici, A.; Roșca, D.; Topor, L.; Barbu, M. Neurovascular Abnormalities in Gartland III Supracondylar Fractures in Children. *Chirurgia* **2013**, *108*, 241–244. [PubMed]
8. Reinstein, L. Hand dominance in carpal tunnel syndrome. *Arch. Phys. Med. Rehabil.* **1981**, *62*, 202–203. [PubMed]
9. Goldberg, C.; Dowling, F. Handedness and scoliosis convexity: A reappraisal. *Spine* **1990**, *15*, 61–64. [CrossRef] [PubMed]
10. Borton, D.; Masterson, E.; O'Brien, T. Distal forearm fractures in children: The role of hand dominance. *J. Pediatric Orthop.* **1994**, *14*, 496–497. [CrossRef] [PubMed]
11. Hassan, F. Hand dominance and gender in forearm fractures in children. *Strateg. Trauma Limb Reconstr.* **2008**, *3*, 101–103. [CrossRef] [PubMed]
12. Mortensson, W.; Thönell, S. Left-side dominance of upper extremity fracture in children. *Acta Orthop. Scand.* **1991**, *62*, 154–155. [CrossRef] [PubMed]
13. Vito, P.; Maria, R.; Gianluca, T.; Ludovico, L.; Claudia, D.C.; Giuseppe, C.; Sergio, A.; Giuseppe, S. Surgical treatment of displaced supracondylar pediatric humerus fractures: Comparison of two pinning techniques. *J. Funct. Morphol. Kinesiol.* **2016**, *1*, 39–47.
14. Ulici, A.; Herdea, A.; Carp, M.; Nahoi, A.C.; Tevanov, I. Nursemaid's Elbow-Supination-felxion Technique Versus Hyperpronation/forced Pronation: Randomized Clinical Study. *Indian J. Orthop.* **2019**, *53*, 117–121.
15. Vito, P.; Andrea, V.; Maria, R.; Annalisa, C.; Pierluigi, C.; Marco, C.; Sara, D.; Gianluca, T. Is supine position superior to prone position in the surgical pinning of supracondylar humerus fracture in children? *J. Funct. Morphol. Kinesiol.* **2020**, *5*, 57.
16. Tevanon, I.; Liciu, E.; Chirila, M.O.; Dusca, A.; Ulici, A. The use of 3D printing in impoving patient-doctor relationship and malpractice prevention. *Rom. J. Leg. Med.* **2017**, *25*, 279–282. [CrossRef]

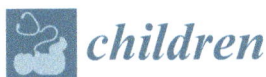

Review

Treatment of Complex Regional Pain Syndrome in Children and Adolescents: A Structured Literature Scoping Review

Andrea Vescio, Gianluca Testa, Annalisa Culmone, Marco Sapienza, Fabiana Valenti, Fabrizio Di Maria and Vito Pavone *

Department of General Surgery and Medical Surgical Specialties, Section of Orthopaedics and Traumatology, Surgery, AOU Policlinico-Vittorio Emanuele, University of Catania, 95123 Catania, Italy; andreavescio88@gmail.com (A.V.); gianpavel@hotmail.com (G.T.); annalisa.culmone@libero.it (A.C.); marcosapienza09@yahoo.it (M.S.); valentifabiana@gmail.com (F.V.); fdimaria95@gmail.com (F.D.M.)
* Correspondence: vitopavone@hotmail.com

Received: 22 October 2020; Accepted: 18 November 2020; Published: 20 November 2020

Abstract: Background: Complex regional pain syndrome (CRPS) is characterized by chronic, spontaneous and provoked pain of the distal extremities whose severity is disproportionate to the triggering event. Diagnosis and treatment are still debated and multidisciplinary. The purpose of this systematic review is to analyze the available literature to provide an update on the latest evidence related to the treatment of CRPS in growing age. Methods: Data extraction was performed independently by three reviewers based on predefined criteria and the methodologic quality of included studies was quantified by the Newcastle–Ottawa Quality Assessment Scale Cohort Studies. Results: At the end of the first screening, following the previously described selection criteria, we selected n = 103 articles eligible for full-text reading. Ultimately, after full-text reading and a reference list check, we selected n = 6. The articles focused on physical (PT), associated with cognitive behavioral (CBT) and pharmacological (PhT) treatments. The combination of PT + CBT shows the most efficacy as suggested, but a commonly accepted protocol has not been developed. Conclusions: Physical therapy in association with occupational and cognitive behavioral treatment is the recommended option in the management of pediatric CPRS. Pharmacological therapy should be reserved for refractory and selected patients. The design and development of a standard protocol are strongly suggested.

Keywords: pediatric; growing age; complex regional pain syndrome; reflex sympathetic dystrophy; multidisciplinary; physical therapy; cognitive behavioral therapy; drugs; pharmacological treatment; occupational therapy

1. Introduction

First described in the 17th century as "causalgia" [1], complex regional pain syndrome (CRPS) is characterized by chronic, spontaneous and provoked pain of the distal extremities whose severity is disproportionate to the triggering event [2]. Three different CRPS subtypes have been distinguished:

- Type 1, previously known as reflex sympathetic dystrophy (RSD), whose cause is not always known.
- Type 2, which results from nerve damage.
- Type 3, or not otherwise specified CRPS, which partly shares clinical and diagnostic aspects with the previous types [2].

CRPS type 1 affects children and adolescents aged 5 to 17 years, with a peak incidence around the 13th year of age, and it is more frequently found in women (70% of cases) [3,4]. The pathogenic mechanism is still unclear, although several hypotheses have been proposed. Genetic factors, altered microcirculation and traumas, such as sprains, fractures and surgical procedures, contribute to pain symptoms. Anxiety, somatization and familial and school problems could also play a role. Chronic pain, generally unilateral and limb localized, autonomic and motor dysfunction and trophic disorders are the main symptoms of CRPS type 1. There are two presentations of the syndrome: the "warm" one, with red, warm, swollen skin that usually occurs in the acute phase, and the "cold" one, with blue/purple, cold, sweaty skin, which is usually associated with the chronic phase [3–6]. The diagnosis of CRPS type 1 is clinical and based on the Budapest diagnostic criteria [4]. However, diagnosis remains challenging due to the lack of validated diagnostic tests and the difficulty of differential diagnosis. Laboratory and imaging tests can be helpful in the event of diagnostic doubt [1]. Treatment is multidisciplinary, and it is mostly based on physical and psychological therapy and medications; only in selected subjects is treatment invasive [7]. The purpose of this systematic review was to analyze the available literature to provide an update on the latest evidence related to the treatment of CRPS type 1 in children and adolescents, highlighting the multidisciplinary approach.

2. Materials and Methods

2.1. Literature Search Strategy

A systematic review of the current literature was conducted according to the Preferred Reporting Items for Systematic Reviews and Meta-Analyses (PRISMA) guidelines [8]. On 20th September 2019, three independent authors (SM, VF and DiMF) performed a systematic review of two different medical electronic databases (PubMed and Web of Science). To achieve the maximum sensitivity of the search strategy, a search string was used ("(complex regional pain syndrome OR reflex sympathetic dystrophy OR Sudeck's atrophy) AND (pediatric OR adolescent OR children OR childhood) AND (treatment OR management)").

2.2. Selection Criteria

The reference lists of all retrieved articles were reviewed for further identification of potentially relevant studies, and the articles were assessed using the inclusion and exclusion criteria. The following inclusion criteria were used when screening titles and abstracts: (a) studies of any level of evidence; (b) studies written in the English language; (c) studies reporting clinical or preclinical results; (d) published studies in peer review journals on the treatment of complex regional pain syndrome type 1. The exclusion criteria were as follows: (a) review articles, (b) case reports, (c) articles written in other languages, (d) diagnosis or differential diagnosis of complex regional pain syndrome type 1. We also excluded all the remaining duplicates, articles dealing with other topics and those with poor scientific methodology or without an accessible abstract. Reference lists were also hand-searched for further relevant studies.

2.3. Data Extraction and Criteria Appraisal

All data were extracted from article texts, tables and figures. Three investigators (SM, VF and DMF) independently reviewed each article. Discrepancies between the three reviewers were resolved by discussion and consensus. The final results and any remaining controversy on the reviewed article were reviewed and discussed with the senior investigators (VA and CA), who served as independent reviewers and assessed study quality. Conflicts about data were resolved by the senior surgeon (PV). Reference lists from the selected papers were also screened. The PRISMA flowchart for the selection and screening method is provided in Figure 1.

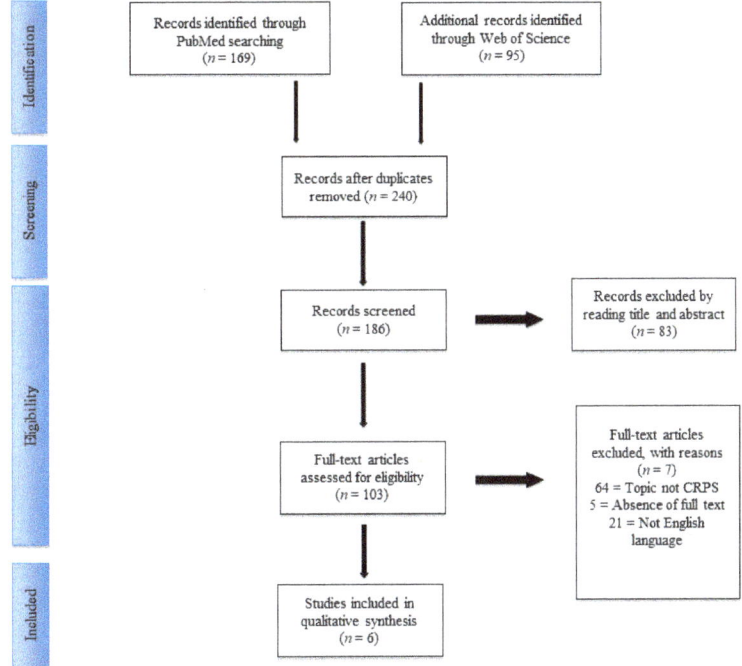

Figure 1. PRISMA (Preferred Reporting Items for Systematic Reviews and Meta-Analysis) flowchart of the systematic literature review.

2.4. Risk of Bias Assessment

A risk of bias assessment of all selected full-text articles was performed according to the Newcastle–Ottawa Quality Assessment Scale Cohort Studies (NOS) [9]. The NOS contains eight items, categorized into three dimensions including selection, comparability and—depending on the study type—outcome (cohort studies) or exposure (case-control studies). For each item, a series of response options is provided. A star system is used to perform a semi-quantitative assessment of study quality, such that the highest quality studies are awarded a maximum of one star for each item, except for the item related to comparability, which allows the assignment of two stars. The NOS ranges between zero and nine stars. The assessments were performed by two authors (VA and CA) independently. Any discrepancy was discussed with the senior investigator for the final decision. All the raters agreed on the final result of every stage of the assessment (Appendix A). In the systematic review, studies classified with more than six stars were included.

3. Results

3.1. Study Selection

From the search of PubMed and Web of Science, 264 articles were included in the review, and 24 studies were selected after duplicate exclusion. Following the inclusion and exclusion criteria, the first screening was performed. A total of 103 papers were considered eligible. Finally, after the full-text reading, reference list check and risk of bias assessment, six studies were included. A PRISMA [8] flowchart of the method of selection and screening is provided (Figure 1).

The main focus of the included studies was related to physical (PT), cognitive behavioral (CBT) and pharmacological (PhT) treatments. A summary of the results is provided in Table 1.

Table 1. Results of selected studies.

Author	Subjects	Dignosis Criteria	Assessment	Treatment	Results	Limits
Brown et al., 2016	Amitriptyine Group: n = 14; Garbapentin Group: n = 15.	Modified International Association for the Study of Pain (IASP) clinical and research criteria.	Coloured Analogue Scale (CAS) Pain 6-weeks post-trial start; Sleep disability as measured on an internally developed 5-point Likert scale; Adverse events.	Amitriptylin 10 mg (at bedtime). Gabapentin at 900 mg/d (300 mg three times per day.	CAS $p = 0.77$. Sleep $p = 0.26$ Adverse events $p = 0.75$.	Small sample size. No randomization. No placebo group. No medium- and long-term follow-up.
Petje et al., 2003	n = 7	Skin examination; burning, dysesthesia, paresthesia and hyperalgesia to cold. Skin cyanosis, mottling, hyperhidrosis, edema and coldness of the extremity and muscles, joint affliction duo to muscle hypotrophy or atrophy and range of motion (ROM) of the joints in the involved extremity. Bonica classification.	Visual analog scale VAS (0–10 points).	Intermittent intravenous infusion of Iloprost at 2 ng/kg/minute for approximately 6 h per day on 3 consecutive days + physiotherapy and psychologic.	VAS = $p < 0.05$. All patients had headache at the first day of infusion. 3 patients had flushing, 2 patients had vomiting. 86% of the sample had a decrease in systolic blood pressure with an average of 7 mm Hg (5–15 mm Hg) in the first 30 min after administration of Iloprost.	No control group Retrospective series. Small number of cases.
Donado et al., 2017	n = 102	Modified International Association for the Study of Pain (IASP) clinical and research criteria.	Preadmission, discharge and 4-month follow-up Pain-Related Functional Disability (PFD) and sleep disturbances (SD) Pain Score (PS).	Continuous regional anesthesia (epidural or peripheral catheter).	PS preadmission median = 7.0; IQR, 5.8–8.2. PS discharge = 3.1; IQR, 1.5–5.4; ($p < 0.0001$). PS 4-month follow-up = 4.3; IQR, 2.0–6.0; ($p < 0.0001$). PFD at admission had a moderate positive correlation with PDF at discharge (r, 0.5; $p < 0.0001$) SD = Yes 48.04%.	Retrospective design. Completed a full course of cognitive behavioral therapy
Logan et al., 2012	n = 56	Modified IASP clinical and research criteria.	At admission and at discharge. Numeric rating Scale (NRS). Functional Disability Inventory (FDI). Lower extremity functional scale: (LEFS). Canadian Occupational Performance Measure: (COPM). Multidimensional Anxiety Scale for Children (MASC). Children's Depression Inventory (CDI). Bruininks-Oseretsky Test of Motor Proficiency, 2nd edition (BOT-2).	Patients participated in daily physical therapy, occupational therapy and psychological treatment and received nursing and medical care as necessary.	NRS = $p < 0.001$ FDI = $p < 0.001$ LEFS = $p < 0.001$ COPM = < 0.001 MASC = $p < 0.001$ CDI $p = 0.003$ All BOT-2 domains = $p < 0.001$. Patients underwent any procedures (e.g., nerve blocks) during or immediately prior to participation in the rehabilitation program.	No randomization. No control group. No isolated treatment effects. Uncontrolled prior treatment history in analyses.

Table 1. *Cont.*

Author	Subjects	Dignosis Criteria	Assessment	Treatment	Results	Limits
Sherry et al., 1999	n = 103	IASP clinical and research criteria.	Visual analog scale (VAS) and Brief Symptom Inventory (BSI) at admission and remission.	An intensive exercise program (most received a daily program of 4 h of aerobic, functionally directed exercises, 1–2 h of hydrotherapy and desensitization). No medications or modalities were used. All had a screening psychological evaluation.	VAS = $p = 0.021$. BSI depression $p = 0.037$. BSI paranoid ideation $p = 0.048$. 1 child (2%) was dysfunctional with CRPS pain, and 5 (10%) had persistent mild pain but were fully functional. Median time between remission of the first episode of CRPS and the start of the second episode = 2 months (range = 2 weeks to 4 years). Predictors of recurrent episodes: previous suicide attempts ($p = 0.026$,), history of an eating disorder ($p = 0.028$).	No long-term follow-up. No control group.
Lee et al., 2002	n = 28. Group A = PT once per week for 6 weeks Group B = PT 3 times per week for 6 weeks.	Wilder et al. criteria.	Pretreatment, at completion of the treatment program and (3) long-term follow-up at 6 to 12 months. Visual analog scale (VAS). Standardized gait impairment score (SGIS), Child Health Questionnaire (CHQ-CF87), Child Depression Inventory (CDI), Revised Children's Manifest Anxiety Scale (CMAS), Compliance.	Individualized physical therapy. Individualized 6 weekly sessions cognitive behavioral therapy. Standard educational program.	At the short-term follow-up, both groups showed improvement in all five outcome measures related to pain and physical functioning ($p < 0.001$ for all measures with a change in median values). There were no between-group differences in any of these measures at baseline or at either follow-up assessment. 79% compliance good.	Small sample. Not standardized after the 6-week protocol.

3.2. Physical Therapy and Cognitive Behavioral Treatment

Three included studies contained a combination of physical therapy and cognitive treatment. Sherry et al. [10] reported the complete resolution of pain symptoms in 74.7% of the sample. Seven subjects did not have remission. One child was dysfunctional with CRPS pain, and five had persistent mild pain but were fully functional. The authors highlighted suicide attempts ($p = 0.026$), an eating disorder ($p = 0.028$), reporting less pain initially ($p = 0.021$) and scoring higher on the Brief Symptom Inventory subsets for depression and paranoid ideation (p 0.037 and 0.048, respectively) as predictors of recurrence. Lee et al. [11] divided patients into two different groups: PT + CBT for 3 weeks vs. PT + CBT for 6 weeks. Both the cohorts showed improvement in all pain and physical functioning outcome measures with short- and long-term follow-up, without differences in pain scores, recurrent episodes of CRPS or participation in school or activities. Logan et al. [12] assessed 56 patients aged 8–18 years at admission and at discharge, and every parameter evaluated had statistically significant improvements. Thirty-two percent of patients required an assistive device at admission, while none required one at discharge.

3.3. Pharmacological Treatment

Petje et al. [13] assessed functional outcome in patients treated with an intravenous infusion of iloprost, a prostacyclin analogue. The drug was administered 6 h per day on 3 consecutive days. Among the side effects noted were headache on the first day of infusion in all patients and flushing and vomiting on the second day in three patients. A decrease in systolic blood pressure of an average of 7 mm Hg (5–15 mm Hg) in the first 30 min after administration was detected in almost the entire cohort. Improvement of the visual analogue scale (VAS) score was found ($p < 0.05$). Relapse of CPRS was experienced by two patients, the first after 3 months. Brown et al. [14] analyzed the outcome of 29 patients refractory to PT + CBT. Fourteen subjects underwent amitriptyline administration, and 15 underwent gabapentin administration. After the 6-week trial, both cohorts showed improvement in pain symptoms, sleep disturbances and functionality. No statistically significant differences were found ($p = 0.77$) between the drugs. Similar adverse events were recorded ($p = 0.77$). Donado and colleagues [15] investigated the use of continuous regional anesthesia (epidural or peripheral catheter) in subjects refractory to PT + CBT. Their data showed significant changes between admission and discharge for pain ($p < 0.0001$), without significant changes throughout the 4-month period after admission ($p > 0.05$).

4. Discussion

According to our data, the physical therapy combined with cognitive behavioral treatment should be considered as the most appropriate first-line approach in CRPS-affected children and adolescents. The pharmacological therapy was found to be efficient in the PT + CBT failure case; the use of drugs is useful only in selected patients subjected to adjuvant physical and cognitive protocol. Nowadays, the lack of comparison treatment studies and specified outcome measurements does not allow for more detailed analysis or the development of a standard treatment.

CRPS is a common but not completely understood disorder, with no available data about the incidence of pediatric CRPS [5] because the diagnosis is uncertain and underestimated. Early diagnosis is as important as treatment; in fact, a longer disease course and sequelae [2] are associated with late identification. Unfortunately, no specific diagnostic tools have been developed for children and adolescents, so the adult criteria are used [5]. Orthopedists have a key role in the recognition of the disease due to very little evidence, no common consensus among the physicians and a lack of guidelines [6]. As reported by Berde and Lebel [16], often, the choice of treatment may vary according to the experience and resources of the clinician. Several treatments have been described [2], including acupuncture, transcranial magnetic stimulation and invasive procedures, but the efficacy has been proven for the combination of physical and cognitive behavioral therapy and only pharmacological treatments. The most established treatment is a program of physical rehabilitation and cognitive behavioral therapy [15]. The goal is to restore normal function, increase the joint motion range and load tolerance and strength and concurrently assist the child in accepting and managing the pain [2].

Different protocols were illustrated in selected studies, highlighting the absence of a standard treatment protocol. Sherry and colleagues [10] suggested aerobic training and progressive resistive exercises, in addition to hydrotherapy, desensitization with towel rubbing, hand massage, textured fabric rubs and contrast baths (2 and 38 °C). During the patient's hospitalization, 5–6 h of daily exercise therapy and 45 min to 3 h of home exercise program (HEPs) were performed. In the Logan et al. trial [12], the patients underwent open-chain and closed-chain activities and an individualized HEP, and each child's functional goals, such as playing a specific sport, were incorporated into the physical schedule. In addition, this multidisciplinary rehabilitation approach addresses the entire pain experience, incorporating desensitization, exposure to feared activities, skills for coping with pain and changes to social responses to pain. Lee et al. [11] designed a protocol including transcutaneous electrical nerve stimulation, progressive weight bearing, tactile desensitization, massage, contrast baths and an HEP. Six weekly sessions of individual CBT incorporating pain management strategies, including relaxation training, deep breathing exercises, biofeedback and guided imagery, were also included. Patient compliance, nurse care and parent treatment programs [17] are crucial to promote successful remission from pain and restoration of functional ability. Despite a rigorous rehabilitation program, Sherry et al. described their patients as a motivated and eager to please sample [10]. Lee et al. [11] recorded compliance varying between 78% and 82%. No adverse events were recorded in the three studies, but the remission rate varied between 79% and 100% [10–12]. Several authors have investigated the role of PT + CBT in pediatric CRPS type 1, especially the brain and neurological changes and treatment action on the central nervous system. Frot et al. found evidence of emotional integration of pain in CRPS patients [18]. Lebel et al. [19] concluded that some changes in the brain persist, especially in the amygdala and basal ganglia, even after symptomatic recovery [20]. Diers et al. [21] demonstrated that behavioral extinction training reduces the emotional involvement in processing painful stimuli and induces a shift to a more sensory-discriminative way of pain processing post-treatment. Kregel et al. [22] emphasize that conservative treatments for patients with chronic musculoskeletal pain may induce both functional and morphological changes in predominantly prefrontal brain regions. For these reasons, non-invasive treatments are often recommended, even in recurrent forms [2,4].

On the other hand, the literature presents evidence of good outcomes after intravenous infusion of drugs and regional nerve blockades. Three pharmacological trials were selected in the study, and different molecules were investigated. Petje et al. [13] assessed the outcome of iloprost intravenous infusion, an analogue of prostacyclin, which induces transitory complete sympathicolysis and avoids the anxiety associated with a lumbar sympathetic blockade. Despite the good rate of response, relevant adverse reactions such as headache, flushing, vomiting and a decrease in systolic blood pressure were recorded in all cohorts; consequently, the same authors do not suggest iloprost as primary therapy. Other drugs proposed for treating neuropathic pain were gabapentin and amitriptyline. The first avoids the release of neurotransmitters acting on voltage-gated calcium channels [23], and the latter neuropathically reinforces the serotonin transporter [24]. Brown et al. compared the two molecules in a refractory PT + CBT schedule. The series revealed that both drugs are effective in reducing pain scores and improving sleep, without significant differences. However, ventricular conduction abnormalities were noted in the gabapentin group, while amitriptyline was linked to QT prolongation, torsade de pointes and sudden cardiac death. For these reasons, the use of both drugs in selected patients and with proper monitoring may be considered. Several invasive options have been proposed, including the use of continuous regional anesthesia with epidural or peripheral catheters, which demonstrate a reduction in pain score and improvement in function score at short- and long-term follow-up. On the other hand, in the Donado et al. series [15], 39% of the sample did not experience clinical improvements in pain symptoms, and 43% had no functional advantages.

Nevertheless, the authors suggested the treatment in addition to an active PT + CBT protocol. All the studies included in the systematic review emphasized the utility of PT + CBT, even when additional approaches were undertaken. The comparison of management with versus without rehabilitation was considered ethically unacceptable [2]; however, the outcome may not be related to a single treatment, and the results have been influenced by conservative treatment even in pharmacologic protocol studies. Future research directions should focus on the identification of disease onset mechanisms and the development of more defined, proper and easy-to-use diagnostic tools.

The design of high-quality, prospective, large-cohort, long-term follow-up studies is strongly encouraged, as is the design of a specific assessment score.

Limits of the study are several and included the heterogeneity of the scores utilized in the objective clinical assessment of the patients. VAS score is an unspecific tool which aims to evaluate the pain, a limited feature of CPRS. At the same time, some authors used more specific scores, such as FDI and PFD, which were not initially developed for CRPS. In addition, due to the challenging diagnosis and long, individual and expensive treatments, studies by Brown et al. [14], Petje et al. [13] and Lee et al. [11] included small size samples, but the described protocols were evaluated with great interest for future prospective use. Moreover, the literature contains limited high-quality studies: despite major randomized prospective studies being included in the review, no control group article or direct comparisons between treatments have been published. The results of drug-related trials could be influenced by different factors, such as longer follow-up after the first or second PT + CBT treatment. The absence of standard protocols and the lack of randomized, blinded prospective trials are the main limits in the comparison of study results.

5. Conclusions

Complex regional pain syndrome in children and adolescents remains a challenge for the physician. The definition is not clear or commonly accepted, and this results in several undiagnosed cases. Despite several diagnostic standards being proposed in adults, no specific diagnostic criteria in growing age patients have been developed and proper treatment is often dependent on the physician's experience and the treatment opportunities. A multidisciplinary approach is mandatory for a good outcome. Main findings of this review are represented by the consideration of physical, occupational and cognitive behavioral therapy as the first-line recommended options in the management of pediatric CPRS; pharmacological therapy can be utilized in failure cases. Unfortunately, the lack of a standard, less stressful and expensive protocol remains the main limit of the methodology. PhT often demands patient hospitalization and is reserved for selected subjects; the adverse events are common but considered as minor complications. Moreover, drugs or other treatments are not considered an alternative to the PT + CBT. To define proper diagnostic criteria, expert multidisciplinary committees as well as standard and commonly accepted guidelines and treatment protocol are essential and strongly encouraged. At the same time, the development of pilot studies for multicenter prospective trials could play a key role in the identification of more satisfactory treatments.

Author Contributions: Conceptualization, G.T. and V.P.; methodology, A.V.; software, F.D.M.; validation, G.T., A.V. and V.P.; formal analysis, A.C.; investigation, F.V.; resources, M.S.; data curation, A.V.; writing—original draft preparation, A.V.; writing—review and editing, G.T.; visualization, V.P.; supervision, V.P.; project administration, V.P.; funding acquisition, V.P. All authors have read and agreed to the published version of the manuscript.

Funding: Received no external funding.

Acknowledgments: Thanks for funding "Open Access" to PIA.CE.RI. of University of Catania.

Conflicts of Interest: The authors declare no conflict of interest.

Abbreviations

Complex regional pain syndrome = CRPS; reflex sympathetic dystrophy = RSD; Preferred Reporting Items for Systematic Reviews and Meta-Analyses = PRISMA; Newcastle–Ottawa Quality Assessment Scale Cohort Studies = NOS; physical therapy = PT; cognitive behavioral therapy = CBT; pharmacological treatment = PhT

Appendix A

Table A1. Risk of bias assessment.

Title	Authors	Year of Publication	New Castle-Ottawa Criteria			Final Evaluation
			Selection	Comparability	Outcome	
Complex Regional Pain Syndrome in Children: a Multidisciplinary Approach and Invasive Techniques for the Management of Nonresponders	Manuel J. Rodriguez-Lopez et al.	2015	★		★★★	Poor quality
A randomized controlled trial of amitriptyline versus gabapentin for complex regional pain syndrome type I and neuropathic pain in children	S.C. Brown et al.	2016	★★★	★	★★★	Good quality
Continuous Regional Anesthesia and Inpatient Rehabilitation for Pediatric Complex Regional Pain Syndrome	C. Donado et al.	2017	★★★	★	★★	Good quality
Continuous Peripheral Nerve Blocks at Home for Treatment of Recurrent Complex Regional Pain Syndrome I in Children	C. Dadure et al.	2005	★★	★	★★	Fair quality
A Day-Hospital Approach to Treatment of Pediatric Complex Regional Pain Syndrome: Initial Functional Outcomes	D. E. Logan et al.	2012	★★★	★	★★★	Good quality
Short- and Long-term Outcomes of Children with Complex Regional Pain Syndrome Type I Treated with Exercise Therapy	D. D. Sherry et al.	1999	★★★	★	★★	Good quality
Spinal cord stimulation in adolescents with complex regional pain syndrome type I (CRPS-I)	G. L. Olsson et al.	2008	★★	★	★★	Fair quality
Treatment of Reflex Sympathetic Dystrophy in Children Using a Prostacyclin Analog	G. Petje et al.	2005	★★	★	★★★	Fair quality
Treatment of Reflex Dystrophy in Children Using a Prostacyclin Analog	G. Petje et al	2003	★★★	★	★★	Good quality
Short- and long- term results of an inpatient programme to manage complex regional pain Syndrome in children and adolescents	G. Cucchiaro et al	2017	★★	★	★★★	Fair quality
Subanesthetic Ketamina infusions for the treatment of children and adolescents with chronic pain: a longitudinal study	Kathy A. Sheehy et al	2015	★★	★	★★	Fair quality
Complex regional pain syndrome in children and adolescents	Kachko et al.	2008	★★	★	★★★	Fair quality
Pediatric complex regional pain syndrome	Low et al.	2007	★★	★	★★★	Fair quality
Physical therapy and cognitive behavioural treatment	Lee et al.	2002	★★★	★	★★★	Good quality
Reflex sympathetic dystrophy in children: treatment with trans-cutaneous electric nerve stimulation	Kesler et al.	1988	★★	★	★★	Fair quality

89

References

1. Chang, C.; McDonnell, P.; Gershwin, M.E. Complex regional pain syndrome—False hopes and miscommunications. *Autoimmun. Rev.* **2019**, *18*, 270–278. [CrossRef]
2. Lascombes, P.; Mamie, C. Complex regional pain syndrome type I in children: What is new? *Orthop. Traumatol. Surg. Res.* **2017**, *103*, S135–S142. [CrossRef]
3. Barrett, M.J.; Barnett, P.L.J. Complex regional pain type 1. *Pediat. Emerg. Care* **2016**, *32*, 185–189. [CrossRef]
4. Rabin, J.; Brown, M.; Alexander, S. Update in the Treatment of Chronic Pain within Pediatric Patients. *Curr. Probl. Pediatr. Adolesc. Health Care* **2017**, *47*, 167–172. [CrossRef]
5. Weissmann, R.; Uziel, Y. Pediatric complex regional pain syndrome: A review. *Pediatr. Rheumatol. Online J.* **2016**, *14*, 29. [CrossRef]
6. Williams, G.; Howard, R. The Pharmacological Management of Complex Regional Pain Syndrome in Pediatric Patients. *Paediatr. Drugs* **2016**, *18*, 243–250. [CrossRef]
7. Xu, J.; Yang, J.; Lin, P.; Rosenquist, E.; Cheng, J. Intravenous Therapies for Complex Regional Pain Syndrome: A Systematic Review. *Anesth. Analg.* **2016**, *122*, 843–856. [CrossRef]
8. Moher, D.; Liberati, A.; Tetzlaff, J.; Altman, D.G.; PRISMA Group. Preferred reporting items for systematic reviews and meta-analyses: The PRISMA statement. *PLoS Med.* **2009**, *6*, e1000097. [CrossRef]
9. Stang, A. Critical evaluation of the Newcastle-Ottawa scale for the assessment of the quality of nonrandomized studies in meta-analyses. *Eur. J. Epidemiol.* **2010**, *25*, 603–605. [CrossRef]
10. Sherry, D.D.; Wallace, C.A.; Kelley, C.; Kidder, M.; Sapp, L. Short- and long-term outcomes of children with complex regional pain syndrome type I treated with exercise therapy. *Clin. J. Pain* **1999**, *15*, 218–223. [CrossRef] [PubMed]
11. Lee, B.H.; Scharff, L.; Sethna, N.F.; McCarthy, C.F.; Scott-Sutherland, J.; Shea, A.M.; Sullivan, P.; Meier, P.; Zurakowski, D.; Masek, B.J.; et al. Physical therapy and cognitive-behavioral treatment for complex regional pain syndromes. *J. Pediatr.* **2002**, *141*, 135–140. [CrossRef]
12. Logan, D.E.; Carpino, E.A.; Chiang, G.; Condon, M.; Firn, E.; Gaughan, V.J. A day-hospital approach to treatment of pediatric complex regional pain syndrome: Initial functional outcomes. *Clin. J. Pain* **2012**, *28*, 766–774. [CrossRef]
13. Petje, G.; Radler, C.; Aigner, N.; Walik, N.; Kriegs, A.G.; Grill, F. Treatment of reflex sympathetic dystrophy in children using a prostacyclin analog: Preliminary results. *Clin. Orthop. Relat. Res.* **2005**, *433*, 178–182. [CrossRef]
14. Brown, S.; Johnston, B.; Amaria, K.; Watkins, J.; Campbell, F.; Pehora, C.; McGrath, P. A randomized controlled trial of amitriptyline versus gabapentin for complex regional pain syndrome type I and neuropathic pain in children. *Scand. J. Pain* **2016**, *13*, 156–163. [CrossRef] [PubMed]
15. Donado, C.; Lobo, K.; Velarde-Álvarez, M.F.; Kim, J.; Kenney, A.; Logan, D.; Berde, C.B. Continuous Regional Anesthesia and Inpatient Rehabilitation for Pediatric Complex Regional Pain Syndrome. *Reg. Anesthesia Pain Med.* **2017**, *42* (Suppl. 4), 527–534. [CrossRef]
16. Berde, C.B.; Lebel, A. Complex regional pain syndromes in children and adolescents. *Anesthesiology* **2005**, *102*, 252–255. [CrossRef]
17. Dickson, S.K. Including Parents in the Treatment of Pediatric Complex Regional Pain Syndrome. *Pediatr. Nurs.* **2017**, *43*, 16–21.
18. Frot, M.; Faillenot, I.; Mauguière, F. Processing of nociceptive input from posterior to anterior insula in humans. *Hum. Brain Mapp.* **2014**, *35*, 5486–5499. [CrossRef]
19. Lebel, A.; Becerra, L.; Wallin, D.; Moulton, E.A.; Morris, S.; Pendse, G.; Jasciewicz, J.; Stein, M.; Aiello-Lammens, M.; Grant, E.; et al. fMRI reveals distinct CNS processing during symptomatic and recovered complex regional pain syndrome in children. *Brain* **2008**, *131*, 1854–1879. [CrossRef]
20. Linnman, C.; Becerra, L.; Lebel, A.; Berde, C.; Grant, P.E.; Borsook, D. Transient and persistent pain induced connectivity alterations in pediatric complex regional pain syndrome. *PLoS ONE* **2013**, *8*, e57205. [CrossRef]
21. Diers, M.; Yilmaz, P.; Rance, M.; Thieme, K.; Gracely, R.H.; Rolko, C.; Schley, M.T.; Kiessling, U.; Wang, H.; Flor, H. Treatment-related changes in brain activation in patients with fibromyalgia syndrome. *Exp. Brain Res.* **2012**, *218*, 619–628. [CrossRef]

22. Kregel, J.; Coppieters, I.; DePauw, R.; Malfliet, A.; Danneels, L.; Nijs, J.; Cagnie, B.; Meeus, M. Does Conservative Treatment Change the Brain in Patients with Chronic Musculoskeletal Pain? A Systematic Review. *Pain Physician* **2017**, *20*, 139–154.
23. Dworkin, R.H.; O'Connor, A.B.; Audette, J.; Baron, R.; Gourlay, G.K.; Haanpää, M.L.; Kent, J.L.; Kranem, E.J.; Lebel, A.A.; Levy, R.M.; et al. Recommendations for the pharmacological management of neuropathic pain: An overview and literature update. *Mayo Clin. Proc.* **2010**, *85*, 3–14. [CrossRef]
24. Kremer, M.; Salvat, E.; Muller, A.; Yalcin, I.; Barrot, M. Antidepressants and gabapentinoids in neuropathic pain: Mechanistic insights. *Neuroscience* **2016**, *338*, 183–206. [CrossRef]

Publisher's Note: MDPI stays neutral with regard to jurisdictional claims in published maps and institutional affiliations.

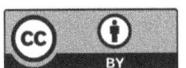
© 2020 by the authors. Licensee MDPI, Basel, Switzerland. This article is an open access article distributed under the terms and conditions of the Creative Commons Attribution (CC BY) license (http://creativecommons.org/licenses/by/4.0/).

MDPI
St. Alban-Anlage 66
4052 Basel
Switzerland
Tel. +41 61 683 77 34
Fax +41 61 302 89 18
www.mdpi.com

Children Editorial Office
E-mail: children@mdpi.com
www.mdpi.com/journal/children

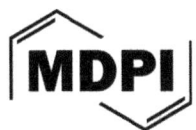

www.ingramcontent.com/pod-product-compliance
Lightning Source LLC
LaVergne TN
LVHW070544100526
838202LV00012B/371